FIT BODY/ FIT MIND

The ABCs of Living Long and Well

By Sharon K. Ferrett, Ph.D.
Sarah A. Bourque, M.A.

Table of Contents

Part One: The Basics of Peak Fitness………………..3

Part Two: The ABC's of Peak Fitness…………….. 13

Part Three: The Practices for Peak Fitness………. 66

Selected Bibliography and Notes

For our husbands, Sam and Ryan. They have made the climb easier and much more fun. We look forward to climbing to the peak and living a long and healthy life. We know the best is yet to come.

"The living self has one purpose only: To come into its own fullness of being; as a tree comes into full blossom or a bird into spring beauty."

--D.H. Lawrence, English novelist, 20th Century

Part One: Introduction

We love the metaphor of life as a mountain. The mountain climber struggles upward, resting at summits and base camps, and then gets up and climbs again. With energy, optimism, passion and focus, the climber forges upward. The struggles and adventures become the journey. During the steep, rocky parts, the climber throws a grappling hook ahead and then pulls on the rope. The peak is the goal, but the joy is the journey. This is how we see aging. It is an amazing mountain that we climb and the steep parts create a challenge and adventure. We climb because we are on the path. We climb because we love adventure and learn lessons along the way. We climb because we are alive.

One of our pleasures is to walk through the beautiful redwood forests or climb 400 feet up the Trinidad Head, which is surrounded by the Pacific Ocean. Both are spectacular trails. It was on one of these hikes a few years ago that we talked about living into old age. We imagined what wondrous inventions there might be and how incredible it would be to hold a great grandchild. What kind of people will we be like if we are lucky enough to live to 100? We want to be healthy, pleasant, kind, calm, loving, independent, contented, and full of life experience. We do not want to be curmudgeons who complained about aches and pains and only talked about the "good ole days." Wouldn't it be nice to grow and mature into a wise old sage? What lessons would my 100-year-old self give me right now for living a long and meaningful life? That vision became the seed for this book.

What if you met your higher self at a ripe old age? What would that wise old sage tell you about what matters most and what principles can help create a meaningful life? How would those principles help you age gracefully? What blessings might be passed on to help you live a healthy, independent and joyful life? Chances are you will live well into your eighties or longer. You don't want to just extend the number of years, but increase the quality and meaning of your life. What you do in your 20, 30, 40, 50, and 60's will determine the quality of your life into your 70 80's and beyond. It is never to late, however, to adapt healthier habits and change your thoughts and lifestyle.

My interest in aging began early. Almost everyone in my dad's family lived long and well. I grew up loving and enjoying my 90-plus year-old aunts and uncles. My Aunt Mabel lived until she was 106 and my Aunt Nellie was 103. My dad died prematurely for his family at 84. My mom was 99-years-old and her sister was 94. I grew up admiring elders for their humor, wisdom and experiences. It was only natural that I fell into working in nursing homes. When I was in college, my friends had part-time jobs in retail or as waitresses. I worked in nursing homes. I have always loved talking with elders and continue to be fascinated by their lives. Even though some people lived a long time, they were in pain or not engaged. Others not only lived a long time, but were physically and mentally active. It became clear that the people who aged well took good care of themselves in their 20', 30's and 40's. They didn't wait until 50 to exercise, eat well and adapt healthy habits. As a university dean, I was involved with senior resources and community outreach services including overseeing a program that worked with Native American elders to restore their language. I also started the first Elderhostel program at Humboldt State University. I had lots of chances to observe and talk with older people and learn their secrets. That became the basis for creating my own program of fitness and for the focus of this book.

After officially retiring from the university, I joined the faculty at the university's OLLI program and offer courses in my favorite topics including memoir writing, forgiveness and aging. I also offer classes at two of our local senior assistant living homes. Over the years, I've interviewed hundreds of elders and talked to many wise sages. From these talks came principles and qualities that I wanted to cultivate. In my office are two bookcases packed with books on aging. I've saved clippings, articles and have attempted to keep up on the latest research concerning aging. When I was preparing for my classes called Peak Aging, I wrote a simple manual for living long and well. This book is the outcome of that class.

In the 1970's Dr. Alexander Leaf wrote an article for *National Geographic* magazine about the world's long-living people. He later wrote the book, *Youth in Old Age*. He studied people who live much longer and healthier than is the norm in our society. Years later John Robbins reviews these long-living people's diet and habits in his books, *Healthy at 100* and *Diet for a New America*. We can learn much from studying long-living people. The Abkhasia people who live in a region within Soviet Georgia, the Vilcabamba who live in Ecuador's Andes mountains, the Hunza people who live in the northernmost tip of Pakistan, and the Okinawa people who live in the southernmost Japanese area of Okinawa all live long healthy lives. I've included simple tips from their diets and lifestyles. Although I've included the latest research on the science behind aging well and examples of proven exercises, this is not the focus on the book. Instead, it is intended to be a primer for simple things you can do every day that will make a big difference in living well.

"There are many tenets of Wholeheartedness, but at its very core is vulnerability and worthiness; facing uncertainty, exposure, and emotional risks, and knowing that I am enough."

-Brene Brown

Why We Wrote this Book

This book has been dancing around in my head for years. I've always been interested in exercise, health and well –being and taught a class at the university on living well at any age. I wrote a first draft of this book to use as a guide. Then I put it away and got busy with a number of other writing projects such as living consciously, overcoming fear, and succeeding in school and at work. It wasn't until my doctor said, "You really should teach a class on how to live well at any age. You are up on the latest research and have developed a program that really works for you. This program could really help others."

I asked my daughter, Sarah, to write this book with me because she has always had a passion for healthy living. Although the focus of this book will be for people over 50, these gentle exercises and strategies are applicable for any age. In fact, the time to plan and create a plan for healthy living should start when you're young. The habits you create in your 20's and 30's will determine how you feel and the state of your health in later years. As anyone in their 60's or 70's will tell you, "The time flies by."

The purpose of this book is to help you build healthy habits that will last a lifetime. We'll review the latest research in health and aging, present a variety of exercise that increase strength, flexibility, and balance and discuss healthy eating. We'll explore a wide range of issues that are practical and some that explore the mystery of life.

We believe we need a new understanding and a creative vision for aging. A hundred years ago, 40 was considered old. Now people are living much longer. My Aunt Mabel lived to be a 106 and my Aunt Nellie was 102. My mom was on her way to 100 and they showed us that aging is not an inevitable downward decline, but can be a continuous inspiring, enjoyable, focused and spiritual awakening and upward climb of self-awareness. The goal is not only to live longer, but also to live active, meaningful, creative, useful, independent, and joyful lives. It's about adding life to your years, not just years to your life. It has been said that life is not measured by the number of breaths you take, but by the moments that take your breath away. You can have amazing joy and happiness at any age. Of course, as we age, we will face inevitable physical and emotional losses. If we only focused on the aches and pain and the loss of good friends, we would have a dismal view of aging. If, however, we shift our perception to our inner life, we will become aware of how it becomes more expansive and richer as we age. You can be more interesting, evolved, intuitive, conscious and dynamic as you age. You can develop empathy and compassion and know how to fully love and forgive others. New ideas, inventions, interests, new friends, spiritual insights, and fresh ideas become important than physical looks, clothes, running a marathon or staying up late. This slight shift in perception can be a huge wake up call.

What really matters in life becomes paramount. There it is front and center. The small stuff falls away and the meaningful becomes clear. "What is my purpose?" becomes the question that is written across our heart. As Carl Jung said, "After fifty, every question becomes spiritual." We have the ability to become spiritual mentors and wise sages to the next generation. We can expand our consciousness and reach our full human potential. We can pass on our hard-earned lessons, values, love, and blessings. As I thought about it, many of the concepts that I had already written about such as overcoming fear, embracing change and transitions, and learning to live with uncertainty all of these applied to aging. Growing old is a gift, a privilege and a wonderful opportunity to come into our own fullness of being. The last third of life can be a time of joy and contentment and even high aspirations. This book was designed to inspire you to be open to new learning, experiences, thoughts and relationships. The best is yet to come! Come with us on this grand adventure and mystery.

"We do not lose heart. Though outwardly we are wasting away, yet inwardly we are being renewed day by day."
--Corinthians 4:16

How to Use this Book

This book was designed to use with a journal or notebook for reflections and exercises. You don't need to read it in a sequential way, but open it at any place. The first step is awareness and acknowledging the reality of your body, mind and spirit. Start by knowing your numbers and health issues. If you haven't had a physical recently, make sure you don't have any issues that may prevent you from exercising. Start all exercises slowly and gently. If you experience any pain, stop. You may feel uncomfortable at times, but you should not feel pain. *The goal of this program is to design an exercise, eating and routine program that works for you. The foundation premise is to live consciously and create a life of purpose, meaning and well-being.* Since the mind and body are intertwined, there will opportunity to reflect and write about where you are now and where you want to be.

Part One is designed to present the more effective exercises to increase strength, flexibility, and balance in just a few minutes a day. You will be encouraged to put together your own exercise program that meets your needs. We'll also discuss healthy eating and strategies that will keep you healthy and active. We encourage you to reflect on what healthy living means to you and explore your fears and beliefs about aging and determine what you want out of life. Add to the list of principles and qualities that you'd like to cultivate.

Part Two is designed to get your writing and doing exercises. As you go through the alphabet, jot down your thoughts, feelings, reactions and associations. This book isn't designed to be read in one setting, but to pick up, read a few lines and share them with others or think about how they relate to you. Open it anywhere. You'll find that some concepts are repeated in different contexts because they are important for healthy living.

Part Three is designed to get you to plan and complete the paperwork necessary to free you from end of life worry and concerns. Buy a simple three ring binder for important documents (living will), health directives, insurance, latest physical and key numbers, vaccinations, and what mediations and supplements you are taking. You can also include poems, quotes, stories, drawings, art, examples of obituaries and memorials and illustrations. I encourage you to keep a journal close by or a simple pad of paper to jot down thoughts and notes to yourself about what you observe, feel, think and reflect about on a daily basis.

Illustrations can help you in looking back and understanding your life. You can draw a mountain or a spiral or a path to illustrate your life as a journey. My favorite illustration is a river since it is a great metaphor for how life meanders, changes course, and twist and turns. Choose an illustration to draw and indicate where your major turning points and transitions. Loss is a major part of every life. What losses did you experience in every decade? What losses were especially painful? What losses were sudden and which ones were gradual? This book will focus on the inevitable losses of the last third of life. But losses are cumulative and each loss builds on previous losses. Looking back at your life and the losses you've endured can help as you face the inevitable losses that come with aging—the lost of friends, loved ones, health, jobs and careers and independence. You can also look ahead with your illustration. What kind of an elder do you want to be? What is important to you now and what do you think will matter most when you're 70, 80, or 90? How do you plan on being as healthy as possible in old age?

Relax and Enjoy

And so, the story goes: *A frantic lion was trying to cross a raging river, but he couldn't swim. He fought the river, charged at it and attacked it with all his might, but instead of controlling the river, he almost drowned. Exhausted he laid down to rest. In this stillness, he heard the river say, "Do not fight an illusion. Do not struggle with what isn't there." The lion woke up, but was confused. The river was still there and he needed to get to the other side. Once again, the river spoke gently, "I am not your enemy. You don't need to push or attack me. I'm just a river. Wake up." The lion became quiet and observed attentively. He watched the river with fresh eyes. He relaxed. Slowly he stepped in and floated to the other side.*

Life is like a river; it doesn't need to be pushed. It flows by itself. Aging is not the enemy. It just is. Instead of fighting time, enjoy it and give thanks for this gift. Resist struggling, denying, or complaining. Embrace your good fortune—you're lucky enough to be aging. Do what needs to be done to allow your life to flow and unfold--gently, fully, and gracefully. Relax and enjoy. Live long and well.

"There will come a time when you believe everything is finished. That will be the beginning."
                    --Louis L'Amour

"Midway this way of life we're bound upon, I woke to find myself in a dark wood, where the right road was wholly lost and gone"
                    --Dante

Life Transitions

The passage into aging is different for everyone. One 8th junior high student said he felt a mixture of sadness and excitement at his middle school graduation. He would enter high school in a few months and knew his childhood was by and large over and he was entering a new phase of life. Most college students say that the transition from high school to college was harder than they expected. Moving away from home, becoming independent and experiencing loneliness was acute and unexpected. Some people have a mild case of melancholy at 30 as they leave their 20's and carefree days. Many people say they had a midlife crisis at 40 when they felt youth slip away. For others, their 50th birthday is a significant transition and they start to feel old. It may hit them that they are no longer middle age. Some people react by trying to recapture their youth. They may make radical changes, and uproot themselves. Some may buy a sports car, shop for a new wardrobe, go on a diet, have an affair, get a face-lift, take up a risky sport, or change jobs. Other people really take stock of their lives and wrestle with what matters most. Some face self-doubts, feel unsettled, disoriented, or depressed. Some people feel both a physical and psychological unrest. The lines from Dante's *Inferno* suggest a dark, unmarked and unfamiliar path. Some people become restless or even reckless. Reality starts to set in and you realize that you're not going to be a college president or the head of your own company. Several other big transitions may occur at the same time. Children may leave for college, the death of a parent or changes in physical endurance or never experienced before pain or illness can all be wake up calls. Other people go inward. This becomes a time of reflection and asking the big questions about life and death. What does this all mean? Did I make a difference in my career? Did I do a good job raising my children? They may start to meditate, take classes, do dream work, read, and ponder their unlived lives. What is it they still want to do? What dreams have been sleeping?

For me, I took note on my 60th birthday. I divided my life into thirds. The first third was spent growing up, going to school and college and getting my first professional jobs in Michigan. The second third was becoming secure professionally, getting married, having children and starting my writing career. The third phase was entering young old age. I started to think about retirement and what I really wanted to do with my last third of living. I didn't feel depressed in the least, in fact, I was grateful that I was still alive as a few friends had died. I felt healthy, passionate about my work, and excited about the last third of life. When I read *The Fountain of Age* by Betty Friedan, I realized that others do not share my optimistic view. She wrote that she felt she was being pushed out of the race professionally and personally. "I could not face being sixty." Some of my friends shared Freidan's ambivalence and even despair about the indignities of old age. While other friends celebrate each year with great joy and thanksgiving. They feel very lucky to have the privilege to grow old.

Starting with the transition of going from junior high to high school, leaving childhood, going away to college or leaving home, settling down with a career and family, reaching mid-life and beyond are all rites of passage and something to pay attention to. When I moved to California, I felt independent and alone for the first time (Sharon). When I spent a year in Italy, my confidence grew and I felt I could take care of myself (Sarah). After my father died, I woke up to the realization that life is short even if you live a long time (Sharon). Regardless of where you are on your journey, transitions and change are part of life. Begin today to make the most of every day.

Life is a gift and one that should not be taken for granted. Erik Erikson wrote about the aging process as tension between the generative period of life and stagnation. Believing that old age means poor health and stagnation is a self-fulfilling prophecy. Because our parents and grandparents were so active and mentally sound, we never saw this slowing down phase as decline, but as a time of expansive inner growth. Perhaps after the shock of turning 60 or 70 or 80 fades, there emerges a time of quiet and reflection and out of that fallow time, a growing appreciation of rebirth into the true fullness of life. Like any major transition, letting go of what was is followed by a shaky wilderness period of confusion and questioning until a new beginning emerges. On solid ground again, it becomes clear that life is a blessing than we could never have imagined when we were young. We can generate kindness, compassion, understanding, empathy and service. When my dear cousin, Ruth, was dying she told me that all she ever wanted to be was a blessing. She was. To bless and be blessed--now that is generating your full humanity. Often this wisdom becomes clear only after we have gone through midlife and enter into old age. The path becomes clearer and we are on a journey with soul. At any age, people do want a life of meaning, but perhaps more important is to feel alive.

What makes you feel alive?

> My fiftieth year had come and gone,
> I sat, a solitary man,
> In a crowded London shop,
> An open book and empty cup
> On the marble table-top.
>
> While on the shop and street I gazed
> My body of a sudden blazed;
> And twenty minutes more or less
> It seemed, so great my happiness,
> That I was blessed and could bless.
> --W. B. Yeats

Questions to Reflect and Discuss

Yeats wrote about an empty cup. Did your cup feel empty as you entered into various transitions? Which one is the hardest to date?
How do you fill your cup?

If your cup is empty, what are your choices? How can this be a blessing?

What do you crave?

What satisfies your hunger and thirst in life?

Do you feel that you have choices that will give you stimulation and satisfaction?

How do you serve and contribute your talents and time?

What does your soul yearn for that hasn't been fulfilled?

How do you bless others? Who blesses you?

How do you cope with change and develop the courage necessary to transcend transitions and move on?

Two Pockets in Your Coat

"Be humble for you are made of Earth.
 Be noble for you are made of stars."
  --Serbian Proverb

   From my observation, it seems really important that elders be respected and honored for their experiences. I feel they have earned the right to speak their truth, express their wishes and find their voice. But at the same time, it seems equally important that they be respectful and concerned about others and not to feel that the world revolves around them. There is a tension between having dignity and self-respect and not being self-absorbed.
   There is an old story from the Talmud that addresses this fundamental human problem of balance between humility and pride.

   Have two pockets in your coat. In the one pocket carry a piece of paper on which is written: "I am but dust and ashes I am but a grain of sand."
   In the other pocket carry a piece of paper on which is written: "For me the world was created!"

How do you carry both of these pieces of paper with you at the same time?

Which piece of paper is bigger?

How do you feel about being humble and noble and the balance between the two?

"To have courage for whatever comes in life—everything lies in that."
  --Saint Teresa of Avil

TAKE TEN

The Best Exercises to do in Ten Minutes

Only have ten minutes or less? This is an example of a core workout that you can vary as you like. I add stretching and balance exercises as well. (see part three).

- 1. promote strength development for all major muscle groups of the body
- 2. use large muscle groups to create the appropriate resistance and aerobic intensity
- 3. create a balance of strength throughout the body (*e.g.*, you would not want to prescribe five exercises for one body part while only prescribing one for another; creating a balance of strength around a joint is an effective way to prevent injury and improve movement efficiency ([1]))
- 4. be immediately modified or adapted as necessary to increase or decrease exercise intensity
- 5. be safe and appropriate for the participants in the training space provided
- 6. be interactive with the available features of the training environment (*e.g.*, stairs, benches, walls, etc.)
- 7. be easily transitioned to accommodate minimized rest time

All exercises can be done with body weight and implements easily acquired in almost any setting (*e.g.*, home, office, hotel room, etc.). The exercise order allows for a total body exercise to significantly increase the heart rate while the lower, upper, and core exercises function to maintain the increased heart rate while developing strength.

Exercises are performed for 15- 30 seconds. Total time for the entire circuit workout is approximately 7-10 minutes. (Illustration in Section Three).

1. Jumping jacks Total body
2. Wall sit Lower body
3. Push-up and rotation.
4. Abdominal crunch Core
5. Step-up onto chair Total body
6. Squat Lower body
7. Triceps dip on chair Upper body
8. Plank Core
9. High knees/running in place Total body
10. Lunge Lower body
11. Push-up and rotation Upper body
12. Side plank Core

Yoga, Tai Chi and Stretching

Start your morning with gentle exercises that tone, stretch and increase your flexibility and balance. Breathe deeply and center yourself. Do a few shoulder rolls, allow your head to drop to each side, do the clock exercise as you reach for the ceiling. Increase your balance with the ABC exercise and balancing on one leg. Exercise your toes and ankles as you lift. Weave in stretching exercises for your spine such as the Cat movement. These will be demonstrated in class.

The Ten Principles of Aging Well

1. **Do Accept Reality**. Physical, mental and spiritual growth comes through acknowledging and accepting reality, rather than ignoring or denying. The way to feel peace and joy is to acknowledge the reality of change. Don't deny or repress your feelings or fears, but be attentive, feel them fully, and question them. "Why is my body changing? Do I fear aging?" Wholly listen and notice with an open mind. Do what you can to make positive change and then relax and enjoy what is. Instead of looking for flaws, faults, and wanting things to be different than they are, focus on the positive. Live in the present moment rather than glorifying the past or worrying about the future. Don't let regret replace your dreams. What is, is. **Don't Whine.**

2. **Do Build Strong Relationships.** Connect with others by knowing your own heart and speaking clearly and with transparency. Communicate in an assertive, respectful, direct and tactful manner. Listen non-defensively. Make friends with people of all ages and appreciate them for their diversity. Honor and value elders for their experiences, wisdom, and contributions. Value the energy and new ideas of youth. Honor the wisdom of elders. Enjoy and listen to children. Appreciate the amazing value of play and fantasy by being with children. Live your life fully and allow others to live their lives. Too often we are blind to our shortcomings, but see then clearly in others. Be aware of projecting your faults onto others. Give up the need to be right. Practice being kind and supportive to all people. **Don't be Critical.**

3. **Do Practice Gratitude**. Live in the present. Give thanks for what you have and for each moment that you are alive. Savor each day with all the simple pleasures and blessings. Be content. Focus on what you have, not what you've lost—or what you've had to give back. Just a slight shift in perception can cause a big shift in consciousness. Focus on love, not fear, abundance, not scarcity, openness, not defensiveness, and acceptance, not struggle. Focus on forgiveness. Forgive yourself for being human and hurting others. Forgive others for hurting you or not living up to your expectations. It really is time to let go of the past. See the humanity in everyone. Let go of slights and real or imagined wrongs. Practice taking less offense, blaming others, and taking things personally. Remind yourself that you are not the target, but the hero. Live in the present moment instead of the past. Sit quietly and allow your blessings to wash over, around and through you.

Don't rehash what could have or should have been. **Don't Focus on the Past or See Yourself as a Victim.**

4. **Do Develop a Sense of Humor.** Have a good belly laugh every day. Watch funny movies, read funny books and enjoy the comics. Learn to laugh at yourself and don't take yourself too seriously. Surround yourself with people who enjoy life. Remember you are not your ways, your thoughts or your opinions. You are much more. Learn to observe your defenses and attachments. Laugh at them. See the humor in every situation. With curiosity and love, look at the ambiguity and the irony of life and of your reactions. Ask, "Where did that self-righteous thought come from? Why did I react as a curmudgeon? Why am I so negative?" Smile. See the humor in being human. Do what you can to make positive change, but don't become a pessimist. The human race has lived through and survived very tough times. Read history and focus on people who made a difference and kept their sense of humor and humanity. **Don't Take Yourself or Life Too Seriously.**

5. **Do get Moving.** Honor your body. Eat consciously. Increase fruits and vegetables, nuts, lentils, beans, fermented foods and lean protein and reduce sugar, additives and processed foods. Listen to your body and exercise! Use all your senses to be in the present moment. Savor your food, smell the flowers, listen to music, dance, sing, and dig in the dirt. Do yoga and Tai Chi. Take walks. Look what you can still do with your amazing body! **Don't be Sedentary or Complain About Aches and Pains.**

6. **Do get Engaged.** Honor your mind. Expand beyond what you know by being open and curious. Be a lifelong learner and allow wonder to enlarge your comfort zone. Explore! Read! Question! Wonder! Listen to different views and opinions. Be a critical and creative thinker. Get engaged. Just remember to stay positive, resourceful, and work for and not against something. Be useful. Find work that is meaningful, fulfilling, and interesting. Make a contribution to making the world a better place. The more involved you are in creating your own happiness, the less demanding you'll be of others. Be attentive to any passion that divides or excludes or demeans others. What is it you came to earth to do? Making a deep creative contribution to your community will help you to feel fulfilled. The world doesn't revolve around you. **Don't be self-centered or accept your opinions as the truth.**

7. **Do Create a Meaningful Life.** Honor your spirit and explore what is most important to you. Find your purpose in life. Focus less on the inevitable physical losses and decline and more on the amazing gifts of time, insights, generosity of spirit, and timeless, enduring and endearing qualities of the spirit. Commit

yourself to key values such as honesty, harmony, responsibility and kindness. The inner life is supposed to become more important with age. Focus on the essence of what unifies humanity and on values that are important for enriching life. Meditate through quiet sitting, centering prayer, walks in nature, or through a regular practice. Find that center of calm and peace and reflect on the mysteries of life and death. When adversity comes, as it will to everyone, respond with courage and creativity. See every challenge as a gift. Breathe deeply. Conscious living is going deeper than your beliefs and opinions. Seek peace of mine and kindness. **Don't Get Sidetracked by dogma or busyness.**

8. **Do Be flexible and open**. Life is change. Embrace transitions and losses by being fluid and flexible. Learn to let go and give up trying to control things that are beyond your control. You cannot control the feelings of others, whether or not people like you, the past or the future. Sometimes you just have to let others live their lives. Do what you can and allow life to unfold. Be open to new ideas and ways of being. Be pro-active and explore creative ways to be independent and to live life to the fullest. Take advantage of all the recourses available in the community. Ask, "How can I see this differently?" Know that you have the ability to adjust and adapt. Improvise. Experiment. **Don't be closed-minded, rigid, or controlling.**

9. **Do Take responsibility.** Own your life and your choices and trust your intuition. As you get older, you may find a knowing in your bones and are less likely to be impulsive. Trust that instinct. Be cautious. Take a deep breath. Don't open the door if you don't know someone. Don't give out personal information on the phone or fall for scams. Consult experts, a trusted advisor, or talk with close family and friends before you act. Listen to your inner wisdom and instincts. If something doesn't feel right, it probably isn't. Ask yourself, "What is going on inside and out at this moment?" **Don't Allow Anyone Take Advantage of You.**

10. **Do Be Authentic.** A meaningful life is authentic and truthful. As you grow older, you realize that you don't need the approval of others, nor do you need to impress anyone. You know who you are and what you want. Speak your truth and express your wishes, ideas and opinions with compassion and kindness. Be yourself. Find and express your creativity and full potential. Relax. You are enough. When you are comfortable in your own skin, it is easier to be interested in and sensitive to others. It's ok to say, "I don't know. I'm sorry. This is why I believe this, but I could be wrong." Authenticity is essential for living the conscious life. False poser comes from control; real power comes from authenticity. Bring out the best in others and support them finding their authentic voice. **Don't Allow Yourself or Anyone Else to be Humiliated or Diminished.**

TAKE TEN

Ten things to add to your diet:

1. **Organic Veggies-especially asparagus, kale, broccoli, cauliflower, artichokes**
2. **Wild salmon (canned is good) and grass-fed meats and eggs.**
3. **Lentils, beans pressure cook to reduce lectins.**
4. **Green tea, coffee (Good source of antioxidants/reduces risk of diseases)**
5. **Fermented foods—sauerkraut, pickled beets & peppers, miso, yogurt, sour dough. Tempeh (fermented soy). Also add Probiotics**
6. **Apples, berries and variety of fruit including greenish bananas**
7. **Sweet potatoes**
8. **Onions and garlic and turmeric.**
9. **Nuts- 2 brazil nuts a day, plus other nuts**
10. **Avocadoes and good fats such as olive oil and dark chocolate**
    On a daily basis, fill your plate with salad, veggies, protein and fruit. However, don't deny yourself treats. Either have a cheat day or eat healthy 80% of the time allowing 20% to enjoy a variety of foods.

Note: *Check to see that your probiotic contains the strain *Bacillus coagulans* such as Schiff Digestive Advantage.
*La Brea Bakery Reserve breads are GMO free and the dough undergoes a fermentation process that removes harmful lectins.

Ten things to avoid in your diet:

1. **Sugar**
2. **Processed foods.**
3. **Lectins loaded carbs such as wheat, brown rice, quinoa. Instead use sorghum, millet, shirataki noodles and rice which are naturally free of lectins and Indian basmati white rice which has very little.**
4. **GMO products. Genetically modified organisms harbor lectins that are new to the human diet. They insert foreign genes into plants to make the plant produce more lectins that enhance its ability to resist insects. Lectins mimic the blood sugar-regulating hormone insulin so they instruct the cells to sore incoming blood sugar as fat and also prevent blood sugar from entering muscle cells. In short, you have cravings and weight gain occurs.**
5. **Soybean oil.**
6. **Corn-fed cattle, poultry, and fish.**
7. **All sodas including diet soda.**
8. **Fruit juices**
9. **Trans oils**
10. **Artificial sweeteners damage beneficial** microbes.

Additional Reading: *The Plan Paradox* by Steven Gundry, M.D.
Four Hour Diet by Tim Ferris

Intermittent Fasting

There is research to suggest that cutting calories or on-and off- fasting may reduce the risk of cancer, Alzheimer's disease, diabetes, and may even lengthen your life. In animal studies, intermittent fasting increases the resistance of cells to various types of stress and disease. The CALERIE Study (Comprehensive Assessment of Long-term Effects of Reducing Intake of Energy) suggest some anti-aging effects and better health indicators such as cholesterol decreased, blood sugar control improved, and inflammatory markers decreased. Some people go on the 5:2 diet. For two days, they eat a 500 or 600 calorie day. Michele Harvie and Tony Howell in *The 2 Day Diet* are researchers at the Manchester Breast Centre in England. Their studies suggest that intermittent fasting for women with breast cancer may enhance the effectiveness of chemotherapeutic drugs by making cancer cells more vulnerable and may protect normal cells from adverse effects of chemotherapy. You can also fast each night for at least 12 hours. I find this an easier method. I stop eating at 6:00 (sometimes by 5) and do not eat again until around 8 or 9. I have a cup of coffee and a slice of apple at 6 and then breakfast at 8. This plan helps me sleep better, I have more energy, and I maintain an ideal weight without having to diet every day.

Get a Good Night's Sleep*Try for seven or more hours)

1. **Unplug at least an hour before bedtime.**
2. **Drink a cup of Chamomile tea early evening and then stop drinking.**
3. **Stick to a routine. Go to bed about the same time every night.**
4. **Brazil nuts, bananas, walnuts have serotonin which is a natural relaxer.**
5. **Take a warm bath.**
6. **Listen to soothing music and do calming stretches.**
7. **Keep your bedroom cool.**

8. Read a little before you fall asleep.
9. Eat an early dinner and don't snack at night.
10. Take a magnesium/ calcium supplement in evening and melatonin.
11. Don't look at the clock if you wake up.

Stress reduction

The stress hormones promote chronic inflammation and inhibit wound healing.

1. Exercise,
2. Meditate.
3. Try Tapping to reduce anxiety and stress.
4. Get enough sleep.
5. Count to ten
6. Breathe and calm down.
7. Practice yoga and Tai Chi
8. Use your senses. Rose essential oil, lavender, peppermint can help calm.
9. Take a walk everyday outdoors. Play, garden and find engaging hobbies.
10. Eat a healthy diet that is rich in vitamins, minerals, amino acids that support serotonin, a brain chemical that contributes to relaxation and sleep.

Be the calming force – breathe and wait for the wave to pass over you. It takes 90 seconds for an emotion to be triggered, to peak and to start to fade, provided you don't do anything to give it oxygen. Remember, you are not your thoughts or feelings. Allow them to float away and choose to act in creative, positive and resourceful ways.

"To attain true inner freedom, you must be able to objectively watch your problems instead of being lost in them...Once you've made a commitment to free yourself of that scared person inside, you will notice that there is a clear decision point at which your growth takes place."

--Michaela Singer, The *Unthethered Soul*

"The most wonderful thing in the world is someone who knows who they are…and knows what they were created to do."

--Rumi

Tapping

Tapping is a natural, simple process that has been proven to reduce stress and help people experience an increased sense of empowerment. Tapping is also known as Emotional Freedom Techniques (EFT) and has helped thousands of people alleviate physical and emotional pain, anxiety, fear and stress. Tapping is using the power of touch to soothe and heal while you affirm positive, calming and resourceful messages to yourself. Tapping can boost your physical and emotional health and help you calm fears, anxiety, grief, and sadness. You can also use it to reduce public speaking anxiety, stage fright, test anxiety, schoolwork, reduce conflicts with parents and siblings and the pressure that comes with being teased, gossiped about or bullied. In other words, tapping can be done anywhere and at any time to give you relief from stress and fear in all areas of your life. With tapping you can change your thinking from negative to positive. Here's how it's done:

First choose a situation that is causing you anxiety or stress. It is important to acknowledge and accept your thoughts and feelings. You are **paying attention** to a problem or issue. For example, "I'm frustrated with my exercise program because I'm not more flexible and don't feel motivated."

1. **Create a statement**. As you tap, say: "**Even though** I'm frustrated and anxious about my lack of exercise, **I love and accept myself**. I will focus on effort and discipline and know **I can choose** to relax, make time and do my exercises consistently." It is important to love and accept yourself even though you acknowledge that you have setbacks. Own your feelings and thoughts, but realize that you don't have to be controlled by them or act in negative ways. You can choose positive options even when you don't feel like it.
2. **Tap on points**. As you say this statement, you are focusing your attention and energy in a deliberate way. *Tap on the side of one hand three or five times (the karate chop point) * Tap on the side of the eye, *under the eyebrow, *under the eye, *under the nose, *the chin, *the collarbone, *under arm and *top of head.
3. **Repeat a few times**.
4. **Tapping takes only a few minutes.** Do it every day and whenever you feel stressed, annoyed, frustrated, discouraged, negative and less than whole. Do the process even when you don't feel like it.

There are many excellent books and resources available on-line about tapping. I recommend the book, *The Tapping Solution* by Nick Ortner.

The First Three Minutes

You can take control of the first three minutes of every day by knowing how to use the whole of your being—non-verbal communication, personal habits, tone, choice of words, style, breathing, and finally stance-- to make a positive and open mindset. The first three minutes of every day sets the stage. The moment you wake up, give thanks that you have another day to love and serve and be whole. Smile, stretch and take a deep breath filling your lungs with energy. As you get up, do the power stance and visualize the universe having your back as you go about your day. This is why ritual and attitude are so important. Tapping can help you pay attention to your feelings and help you love, accept, soothe and comfort yourself even when you have negative thoughts or issues.

Write out how you start your day to create positive energy and joy.

PART TWO

The ABC's of Peak Aging

"He who knows others is wise,
He who knows himself is enlightened."
    --Lao Tzu

"There is a fountain of youth. It is in your mind, your talents, the creativity you bring to your life and the lives of people you love. When you learn to tap this source, you will truly have defeated age."
    --Sophia Loren

"Far away there in the sunshine are my highest aspirations. I may not reach them, but I can look up and see their beauty, believe in them, and try to follow whee they lead."
    --Louisa May Alcott

"For inside all the weakness of old age, the spirit, God knows, is as mercurial as it ever was."
    --May Sarton

"Who are you? It's an unanswered question, but let us still believe in the dignity and importance of the question."
    Tennessee Williams

"The privilege of a lifetime is to be who you are.

    --Joseph Campbell

A

A is for **acceptance**. Peak aging starts with accepting loss and limitations. You are growing older each day and that means changes both physically and emotionally. If you argue with reality, you always lose. Instead, **acknowledge** your fears and shake your ambivalence about life. It is worth living fully.

Attitude is everything. It is your attitude, more than any other factor, which influences how you experience life. Aging is not the problem; it's your attitude about aging that creates your state of mind. Focus on the best that aging has to offer—the broader perspective, the hard-won wisdom, the serenity, sound judgment, time for yourself, and self-knowledge. Shift your perception to all the good things in your life and the wonderful person you've become and are becoming. **Accentuate** the positive and **appreciate** your life.

Authentic. The most wonderful aspect of growing older is the opportunity to discover your authentic self. You are more than your role as spouse, parent, friend, sibling or community member. You are not your job, body, achievements, beliefs, thoughts, feelings or opinions. You are ageless and formless. Your essence is pure consciousness. You can't think your way to being real, but you can step into the light. Find your voice and express yourself. Grow into your true fullness of being.

Amends. We all have been hurt and have hurt others, but we often have the opportunity to make amends. Try and right the wrong.

Awaken to the wonders of each moment. Become **aware** of the birds singing, children laughing, the morning light, a good meal, companionship with family and friends and the beauty of flowers. Find a tree that calls for your **attention** everyday. Notice the changes and the beauty of every season; fall leaves, winter bareness, spring buds and summer greenness.

Adapt. You must be bold and adaptable to survive old age. Move beyond your comfort zone, change what you can and be willing to try new things. The key is to adapt to what is and make the best of every situation.

Make each day count by being **adventuresome** and being **attentive.**

"What lies behind us and what lies before us are tiny matters compared to what lies within us."
--Oliver Wendell Holmes

"Let the beauty we love be what we do."
--Rumi

"To accomplish great things, we must live as if we're never going to die."
--Luc de Clapiers

"Don't forget until too late that the business of life is not business, but living."
--B.C. Forbes

"Believe that life is worth living and your belief will help create the fact."
--William James

B

B stands for **balance**. Prevent falls by developing good balance, flexibility, and strength with exercise, Tai Chi or yoga. Get a **bone density test** and follow suggestions to increase prevent bone loss and balance.

B**alance** work, play, interests, rest, exercise, and spiritual growth. The most important job in the last third of life is to become more aware, create deep meaning, explore the mystery of life and death, and learn to love yourself and others. This requires contemplative quiet and life review. Beware of the distraction of being busy that can keep you from looking within. Look for patterns that have distracted you in the past.

Breath deeply. Before reacting, use the power of breath to help you respond in an appropriate and calm manner. Breathing deeply, from your abdomen, increases lung capacity, helps with digestion and eases pressure on the spine. Breathing deeply also allows anger to move through you as you remain centered. Change positions often as you breathe deeply.

Beliefs. What are your beliefs and feelings about old age? Too many people have a loathing of growing old and deep-seated fear about death and dying. They surround themselves with other complainers or people who deny they're growing older and try to act and look younger. You can either focus on the belief that aging is a downward spiral of physical decline--wrinkled skin, aches and pains, loss of vigor and waning energy or you can focus on the belief that aging is an upward spiral of expanded consciousness, self-knowledge, experiences, curiosity, wisdom, and a deep sense of meaning, peace, and contentment.

What's on your **bucket** list? What is it you have always wanted to do but have been putting off? Start your list. **Believe** in yourself.

Being. Sometimes just b**eing** is enough. **Be** present.

"It is better to light one small candle than to curse the darkness."
                        --Confucius

"Complacency is the enemy of study. We cannot really learn anything until we rid ourselves of complacency."
                      --Mao Tse-Tung

"All doors open to courtesy."
                      --Thomas Fuller

"Character makes flesh and blood comely and alive; it adorns wrinkles and old hair."
                      --Yehudi Menuhin

C

C stands for being **connected**. Relationships are the heart of life and become more important as we age and become aware of what matters most. It is important to stay in contact and commit yourself to family and friends. It is important to build new friendships of different ages. **Communication** is the key to loving and authentic relationships. Get involved with groups and service organizations. **Care** about people and your **community.**

Clarity. Be **clear** about what you want and make certain that everyone understands your wishes and end-of-life desires. Almost no one wants to end up in a nursing home, but thousands of competent elders languish in institutions surrounded by strangers because of unclear communication, wanting to be nice, avoiding conflict, or not wanting to be any bother or trouble. Many family conflicts could have been avoided if the aging parent were transparent about wishes, contents of documents and where they are located. There should be no confusion as to how you want to live, grow old, and die. Communicate in a clear, direct, assertive, kind and tactful manner.

Complaints. You don't want to e a curmudgeon, grouchy, or complaining, about aches and pains. However, be willing to say what you mean and mean what you say. You don't want to be silenced or grow complacent. Be interested, interesting, involved, and real.

Consideration. Just because you are growing older does not give you the right to be rude or inconsiderate. Courtesy, respect, good manners and tact are important throughout life. Create yourself anew daily.

Congruence. When your behavior and choices are in harmony with your values, purpose and inner moral compass, you live an authentic life.

Choice. Each time you face a loss, you have a choice. You can either accept reality or you can deny, evade, struggle, and bury your pain. **Choose** life.

Clutter. If it isn't useful, beautiful, or special, get rid of it. Declutter!

Curiosity will keep you young.

Creativity is important all your life. Just get up everyday. Get going and wear **comfortable** shoes. Take **control** of your life.

Chi Gong is an ancient Chinese health practice that combines gentle movement, breathing techniques and focused intention.

The serenity to accept the things I cannot change and the wisdom to know the difference.
       -The Serenity Prayer

"No one expects the days to be gods."
      --Emerson

"It's not the length of life, but the depth of life."
      --Ralph Waldo Emerson

"I am convinced that it is not the fear of death that haunts our sleep so much as the fear that our lives will not have mattered."
      --Rabbi Harold Kushner

"Death is not the greatest loss in life. The greatest loss is what dies inside us while we live."
      Norman Cousins

D

D stands for **disputing** negative thoughts and beliefs. Ask yourself, "Is this true? How do I act when I believe these thoughts and beliefs? How would I act if I had more loving and kinder thoughts and a positive attitude? Is there another way of looking at this situation? Can I calm my judgmental thoughts long enough to listen to other viewpoints? Can I be open to change and not cling to what was?

Dare. Dare to be the wise, kind, generous, magnificent person you are. Dare to step up and be genuine and vulnerable. Try new experiences. Dare not to be perfect. Dare to speak up. Don't allow anyone to silence you. Share your thoughts, views, joys, sorrows and lessons you've learned. Make your voice known. You no longer need to please or cave into peer pressure. Be a critical and creative thinker who is open to new information, asks questions and is comfortable with not knowing the answers. Dare to change your mind and admit your wrong sometimes. Dare to nurture the virtues of kindness, generosity, compassion, empathy, and creativity. Dare to grow into a wise old sage.

Depth. When young, there is a tendency to skate along the surface; enjoying a wide range of interests, friends and juggling many tasks. Now is the time to go deeper and explore the depth of feelings, ideas, relationships, forgiveness and life itself.

Dignity. Maintain self-respect and respect for others. No one should humiliate you, treat you as a child, or be dismissive of your wishes. Tell people what you'd like to be called, ask them to talk with you directly, and do not allow others to silence your voice or talk down to you.

What kind of a **death** do you envision? What can you do to die consciously and with **dignity?**

There is often a **disconnect** between your actual age and the age you feel. If you're young at heart, get going with your **dreams.**

"Flatter me, and I may not believe you. Criticize me and I may not like you. Ignore me, and I may not forgive you. Encourage me, and I will not forget you."

--William Arthur Ward

"The most exhausting thing in life is being insecure."
--Anne Morrow Lindbergh

"Who is the holy person? The one who is aware of others' suffering."
--Kabir

"Exercise, exercise, exercise. It's the only wonder drug we have."
--Dr. Rosanne Leipzig, Mount Sinai School of Medicine

"If you can't fly, then run. If you can't run, then walk. If you can't walk, then crawl. But whatever you do, keep moving."
--Dr. Martin Luther King, Jr.

E

E stands for **exercise**. If there's a fountain of youth, it's exercise. Get moving! Check with your doctor about the best plan for you. If you're not active, work up slowly to an hour a day. Stand and sit **erect.**

Essence. The core of your being is your soul, the divine, your true and higher self. **Explore** within and see beyond the mundane to the powerful energy field and potential of your inner being. When your actions are congruent with your values and highest aspirations, you experience harmony and peace. Peak aging is simply returning to your true essence, which is pure love. You are far more than your limited roles or l accomplishments. There is an inner beauty and peace so vast and spacious, it will take your breath away. You don't have to strive, struggle, or follow some special path. You just have to be still and awaken. Sit quietly. Meditate and develop mindfulness. **Expand** beyond what you know.

Explore the great mysteries of life and death. **Engage** in life.

Encouragement. At every opportunity, encourage others and lift them up. Criticism doesn't help improve relationships.

Embrace the great mysteries of living and dying. **Embrace and enter** into your grief and trust that you will be transformed. Acknowledge your sorrow and the pain of others. Practice compassion and see the perfection in everything and everyone? Embrace the whole of life.

Empathy. Knowing we are all one, seek to understand and relate to each other. Check your **ego** and listen with compassion.

Eat slowly and consciously. Focus on eating lots of fruits and vegetables, healthy fats, lean protein, nuts, beans, and whole grains. Increase your fiber. Drink more water. Eliminate soda, fast and processed foods.

"Everything has two handles, one by which it can be borne and one by which it cannot. If your brother sins against you, don't take hold of it by the wrong he did you but by the fact that he's your brother. That's how it can be borne."

--Epictetus

"The strongest have their moments of fatigue."
--Nietzsche

"Doing an injury puts you below your enemy;
Revenging one makes you but even with him;
Forgiving it sets you above him."
Benjamin Franklin

"If you do not wish to be prone to anger, do not feed the habit; give it nothing which may tend to its increase. At first, keep quiet and count the days when you were not angry: 'I used to be angry every day, then every other day: next, every two then every three days.' And if you succeed in passing thirty days, sacrifice to the gods in thanksgiving."
--Epictetus

"Reversing your treatment of the man you have wronged is better than asking his forgiveness."
--Elbert Hubbard

F

F stands for **flexibility**. Peak aging requires that we be willing to grow, change and relax. Learn to expect the best, but adapt to what is with a sense of humor and good will. Since you don't know what is best, flow with what is. See life as an adventure like climbing a mountain. You may prefer your nice, warm bed, but you can sleep in a tent for a few nights, eat food you normally wouldn't eat, listen to new sounds, push your endurance and put up with a few aches and pains. It's an adventure and you know how to flow with life. You've learned that being rigid and fixed in your thinking creates an old, cranky person who finds fault with everything. Adapt. So your daughter is late, your grandkids don't send you thank you notes, the server at the restaurant is busy and you have to wait longer than usual. So what. Be flexible. Relax. Find that place of calm, peace and joy within. Life is good.

Friends. Make time to find and appreciate kind, gentle, positive, interesting, supportive and loyal friends of all ages. Although you may be more comfortable with people who share the same views, learn to listen and appreciate people who come from a different culture, religious, racial, political background and have different experiences or viewpoints than you. Empathy and understanding can open up a new world.

Forgiving. It is so important to forgive yourself and others. The burden of not letting go of the past will eat away at your soul. Make amends whenever possible, say you're sorry, and allow grievances to fall away. The past is over. Forgive yourself and others. Heal misunderstandings.

Fears. The greatest fear of many is to be useless, idle and invisible as they age. There is also the fear of loss, dying, and all the unknowns. Aging is a natural process and becoming more open and knowledgeable about aging, death and dying can help overcome these fears. Go to the library and start your education. Explore new possibilities and rethink your idea of work, success, and contribution. Enjoy the slower lane as you engage.

"That man is happiest who lives from day to day and asks no more, garnering the simple goodness of life."
\qquad --Euripedes

"If the only prayer you say in your whole life is 'thank you,' that would suffice."
\qquad --Meister Eckhart

"Gratefulness is the gallantry of a heart ready to rise to the opportunity a given moment offers."
\qquad --David Steindle-Rast, Gratefulness, the Heart of Prayer

"Men often bear little grievances with less courage than they do large misfortunes."
\qquad --Aesop

"Most humans have an almost infinite capacity for taking things for granted."
\qquad --Aldous Huxley

"The great use of life is to spend it for something that outlasts it."
\qquad William James

G

G stands for **gratitude.** Appreciating and giving thanks for all your blessings is a way to transform your life. It's as if the world is suddenly full of color, light and sound. Gratitude creates an upward spiral of energy that attracts abundance in all forms. Breathe in the beauty and simple goodness that is all around you. Take nothing for **granted.** Appreciate good friends, food, flowers, books and give thanks.

Grief. It is important to grieve for all your losses and feel all your emotions fully. It is hard to lose loved ones, difficult to lose physical stamina, recognition, youthful looks, jobs, and a feeling of usefulness. When you have observed and fully accepted your feelings of grief, allow these emotions to flow through you and over you. Watch them float away like clouds. Your mind is so vast and your heart is so spacious, it can hold many thoughts and feelings. You do not have to stay stuck in suffering. Breathe deeply and allow them to float away.

Generosity. Be generous with your time, love, praise and attention.

Grievances. You cannot live a full and happy life if you're holding on to grievances. What little annoyances cause you a lack of peace?

Goals. What is it you want? How do you want to live? What are your goals? My goal is to be useful, strong, fit, engaged, loving and beloved.

Gaia is the living planet earth. How do you view your place in the universe?

Being a good person is more important than achievements. Live an ethical and morally sound life.

"When health is absent
Wisdom cannot reveal itself,
Art cannot become manifest,
Strength cannot be exerted,
Wealth is useless, and
Reason is powerless."
                    --Herophilies, 300 B.C.

"Perhaps one has to be very old before one learns how to be amused rather than shocked."
            --Pearl S. Buck

"The best and most beautiful things in the world cannot be seen or even touched. They must be felt with the heart."
                    --Helen Keller

"None so deaf as he that will not hear."
        Thomas Fuller

"Of all feats of skill, the most difficult is that of being honest."
        Marie De Beausacq

Katy Butler says that three quarters of Americans say they want to die at home but only a quarter do. Two-fifths of all deaths now take place in a hospital and a fifth happen in ICU's.
        Katy Butler, *Knocking on Heaven's Gate*

H

H stands for good **health**, which is fundamental for living long and well. If you have your health, you have everything and anything is possible. Many problems that are considered to be part of aging can be eliminated with healthy habits. To be healthy, you've got to get moving and be conscious of what you're eating. This principle is hard until it isn't. Once you make a ritual out of daily exercise and conscious, healthy eating, it becomes a habit that you simply do everyday. Keep it simple. Eat more veggies and fruit, nuts, whole grains, and eat less processed foods. If you need to lose weight, eliminate anything made with flour and sugar. It works. Take the stairs. Walk more each day until you're exercising for about an hour *every day*. Really. That's what it takes for peak aging. Then add weight bearing exercise and take Vitamin D plus get about ten minutes of sunshine to keep your bones healthy and strong. Get a check up every year and ask your doctor how you can be healthier. Don't smoke, overeat or drink to excess. Get the shingles vaccination if you're over 50. If you are healthy, you are attractive and young looking because vitality overshadows the normal signs of aging. It's not that complicated. Eat less, exercise more, eat real, whole food and reduce stress.

Humor. Being able to laugh often is key to staying young. Learn to find humor in almost every situation. Take yourself less seriously.

Heart. Critical thinking is important and so is listening to your heart and intuition. Sometimes you just know that something is the right thing to do. Put more emphasis on matters of the heart rather than material things. Expand your heart to be more generous with support, time and understanding.

Help others. Help your aging parents, neighbors, volunteer at an assistant living. It will help you develop patience, empathy and compassion.

Hope is essential. The human spirit is resilient and creative. Work for making the world a better place, with **hope, hard work**, and optimism.

If you want to die in your own **home**, plan ahead.

Hydrate. Drink water and tea throughout the day.

"Good intentions are useless in the absence of common sense."
 --Jami

'A long life may be good enough, but a good life is long enough."
 --Benjamin Franklin

"It is not the years in your life but the life in your years that count."
 Adlai Stevenson

"Very truly, I tell you, when you were younger, you used to fasten your own belt and go wherever you wished. But, when you grow old, you will stretch out your hand, and someone else will fasten a belt around you and take you where you do not wish to go."
 --John 21: 18

"I am done with great things and big plans, great institutions and big success. I am for those tiny, invisible loving human forces that work from individual to individual, creeping through the crannies of the world like so many rootlets, or like the capillary oozing of water, which if given time, will rend the hardest monuments of pride."
 --William James

"The essence of age is intellect."
 --Ralph Waldo Emerson

I

I stands for **independence**. Everyone wants to be independent as long as possible. It is a national shame that elders are warehoused or institutionalized in nursing homes instead of revering them with honor and dignity. In most cases, elders can age in place in their own homes with smart planning. Good health is the first place to start. Invest in it early to prevent later problems. Learn how to be responsible for yourself. Married people often fall into roles and are lost when a spouse dies. Make certain you know how to pump gas, pay the bills, make repairs, cook, clean, wash clothes, turn off the water, garden and all the other tasks that make up a life. Occasionally, do things on your own. Take small trips, have lunch or dinner out, go to a movie. It's more fun to be with a spouse, companion or friend, but it is also good experience to do things on your own occasionally. Get help before you need it. If you're alone, consider renting out your room to another person or if needed a nurse or aide. Do what you can to stay independent.

Involvement. Although you want to strive for balance, you also want to be involved in your community. It makes your life richer when you have communities such as a church, politics, service groups, book clubs, dining, bridge, garden railroad, dog agility, etc. Find a project that engages your passion, time, and energy.

Age is **irrelevant.** How do you feel? What do you love to do? As long as you're **interested** in life, you're young at heart.

Invisible. What is invisible to the eye, but is essential to your life? When did you learn the truth about this?

Your **inner self** or spirit now has the opportunity to come into its true realization. Do meditation, dream work, quiet reflection and tackle all the great mysteries of life. Listen for clues and happenings that point the way.

"You cannot be too gentle, too kind. Shun even to appear harsh in your treatment of each other. Joy, radiant joy, streams from the face of one who gives and kindles joy in the heart of one who receives."

--St. Seraprum of Sarov

"The jealous are troublesome to others, but a torment to themselves."
--William Penn

"What you see in others has more to do with who you are than who other people are."
--Eictetus

"The mere sense of living is joy enough."
--Emily Dickenson

J

J stands for **judgment**. It is a hard lesson to learn, but important: no one likes to be criticized. Separate your business, other's business and the universe's business. How your daughter keeps her house is not your business. How your son spends his money is not your business. Natural disasters, death and other biggies are way beyond our worry or control. Focus on what you can do to improve yourself and what is clearly your business. Learn to be more open and rest easier with ambiguity. Most of the time, we simply don't know. Things are often not what they seem so our opinions, beliefs, intentions, and criticisms are usually not true and rarely helpful. Judging is exhausting and unnecessary. You also save a lot of time when you're not labeling, evaluating, and interpreting. Use all this extra time and space in your head to simply enjoy life.

Joy. When you are at peace with yourself and life, your natural state of joy bubbles up. It is who you are. Be kind and gentle with yourself and others and you will feel your joy.

Jealousy. Being happy for other's successes and achievements is one mark of an emotionally mature person. View even a small tinge of jealousy as a kick in the rear to get going and find your passion. Be useful and productive and you won't have time to envy others.

Join with others in fellowship. Find your tribe in hobbies, church, taking classes or other interests groups.

Keep a **journal** of notes, thoughts, reflections, memories, ideas, favorite stories and daily events.

Life is a **journey** and the reason you're still here is that you still have something important to do on your path. What is your life's purpose?

Juggle your schedule so you have time for loved ones, time to work and serve and time for quiet and stillness and reflection.

"Life is just a short walk from the cradle to the grave—and it sure behooves us to be kind to one another along the way."
> --Alice Childress

"Kindness is the language which the deaf can hear and the blind can see."
> --Mark Twain

"I expect to pass through life but once, If, therefore, there be any kindness I can show, or any good thing I can do for any fellow being, let me do it now…as I shall not pass this way again."
> --William Penn

"Assuredly, I say to you, inasmuch as you did it to one of the least of these My brethren, you did it to Me."
> --Mathew 25:40

"The knower and the known are one. Simple people imagine that they should God as if he stood there and they here. This is not so. God and I, we are one in knowledge."
> --Meister Eckhart

K

K stands for **kindness**, which becomes more important every year. It is entertaining and fun to be around someone witty, clever, intelligent and cultured, but kindness is more important than all the witty comebacks. Cultivate the kindness within you. Your friends and grandchildren don't care a wit if you have wrinkles, but they yearn for a gentle, kind, understanding, and loving spirit to be present.

Let others be **kind** to you. Accept help and small acts of kindness. Don't resent it when people offer to assist you. It is easier for a happy person to be **kind** and a kind person to be happy.

Knowledge. If there is a community college or university close, check out classes. You could finish your degree, get an advanced degree or enjoy classes through extended education. You might want to study the Civil War era, learn to write your memoir, take a course on geology or learn about gardening or bee-keeping. Be knowledgeable about all the resources in your community. Before you need a service, be aware of what is available. Call your local senior resource center and check out all their programs and services or consider being a volunteer. Ask for help when necessary and be creative when solving problems.

Knowing your style and what looks good on you is more important than the latest fashion. Wear what is comfortable and age appropriate.

No time for **kvetching.**

Keep at it. You never know when some wonderful opportunity, an adventure, a new passion will come along.

"Someday after mastering the winds, the waves, the tides and gravity, we shall harness for God the energies of love. And then for the second time in the history of the world, man will have discovered fire."
--Pierre Teilhard De Chardin

"The world is too dangerous for anything but truth and too small for anything but love."
--William Sloan Coffin

"The most wasted of all days is one without laughter."
--e.e. cummings, American poet

"What matters most is that we learn from living,"
Doris Lessing

"I like living. I have sometimes been wildly, despairingly, acutely miserable, wracked with sorrow, but through it all I still know quite certainly that just to be *alive* is a grand thing."
--Agatha Christie

"The great tragedy of life is not that men perish, but that they cease to love."
--W. Somerset Maugham

"The heart that loves is always young."
--Greek proverb

"A cheerful heart is good medicine."
--Solomon

L

L stands for **listening**. Relationships are built on love and communication and listening is the foundation for connecting. Focus on what the person is saying—not just the words, but also the emotions behind them. Listen with compassion and empathy. Be authentic and gently give your opinion when asked. Don't just parrot back what you think the person wants you to say. Real listening requires understanding and honesty. Sometimes your mind may race ahead when someone is talking. Take a deep breath and practice being calm, focused, and centered on the conversation. If distracted, take a moment to deal with the issue and then go back to the conversation fresh. Listening takes a lot of energy.

Love. Love your work. Love life Don't walk around feeling offended, defensive, angry or guilty. Feel all your emotions, dispute irrational thoughts, and move on. Life is too short not to love yourself and others.

Love learning. Read widely. Become a lifelong learner.

Laugh. We all like to be around people who have a sense of fun, laugh easily and just plain enjoy life. See humor all around you. Laugh at yourself. Don't worry about the small stuff. Laugh every day.

Letters of love will be a gift that your family will cherish. Take time to slow down, reflect and create space for writing. Will your great-grandchildren be impressed that you were on many boards or would they prefer a memoir, lessons you want to pass on, or a simple letter of love from you?

Life is too short to carry around anger and resentment. Forgive.

It is a **luxury** to grow old.

Listen. Your body is speaking.

"When you develop mindfulness and introspection well, you are able to catch laxity and excitement just before they arise and prevent their arising."
    --Dalai Lama

"The world is chock-full of interesting and curious things. The point of courtship---marriage—is to secure someone with whom you wish to go hand in hand through this source of entertainment, each making discoveries, and then sharing some and merely reporting others."
    --Judith Martin (Miss Manners)

"Let there be spaces in your togetherness and let the winds of the heavens dance between you."
    --Kahlil Gibran

"How lucky I am to have something that makes saying goodbye so hard."
    --A.A. Mine
    Winnie the Pooh

M

M stands for **mindfulness**. Focus on one thing and you'll be more effective. Many accidents happen when you're distracted and not aware. If you're walking, walk. Be mindful of each step. Look around and watch for steps or uneven ground. Don't just step out or step back without being mindful of your surroundings. When you are in the moment, centered and calm, you act deliberately and with purpose.

Motivation. Life is a series of transitions each requiring that we ask, "Who am I? What do I want? What are my talents and interests? How can I create meaningful work? How do I get off the dime and get motivated to follow my path?

Meaning. Whenever you invest time, energy, and commitment into a relationship, job or project, you create meaning. When you lose a deep attachment to someone or something, you will experience grief and a sense of loss and purpose. Look at your major life losses. What is the meaning of these losses?

Tell me about **marriage**. What has it meant to you?

Doing creative exercises, reading and changing your routine can enhance **memory**. For example, brush your teeth, hold the phone, write and eat with the hand you don't normally use. Do crossword puzzles or math.

Be a **mentor.** Pass on your experiences, knowledge and wisdom.

It is **magical.** The more your give of yourself, the more you gain.

Map out the last third of your life. On a sheet of paper, sketch out alternative paths. What is the true version of your life? Reflect on possibilities. You can always change your mind or go to plan B.

Move. We evolved to **move and exercise.** Get going!

"In the hope of reaching the moon men fail to see the flowers that blossom at their feet."
--Albert Schweitzer

"It is never too late to be what you might have been."
--George Eliot, English novelist

"All men should learn before they die what they are running from and why."
--James Thruber

A human being fashions his consequences as surely as he fashions his goods or his dwellings. Nothing that he says, thinks or does is without consequences."
--Norman Cousins

N

N stands for **notice**. Notice the beauty of a flower, a grain of sand, the laugh of a child. Practice noticing with curiosity, clarity, and a sense of wonder. Observe what is going on within you and around you. Be aware. If something doesn't feel right, trust your intuition. When you walk to your car after buying groceries, notice your surroundings. Be prepared. Get your keys out, have your purse in front of you, not daggling from your shoulders. If you don't feel comfortable, ask a clerk to help you with your groceries. Lock your car when you get inside. If you're like many people, you may be in a daze or thinking about dinner tonight rather than the safety of your surroundings. When you look distracted, lost, or fumbling, you look vulnerable and robbers can pick you out of a crowd as an easy victim.

No. Say "**NO**" to negative thoughts, patterns and behaviors. Notice and allow them to float away. Don't let your chattering mind take off and create a grievance story.

Nature. Get outdoors and enjoy nature. If you live in the city, go to parks and nature preserves. Go to the country as often as possible to breathe in fresh air and to observe, listen and take in nature.

Nurture intimacy with your spouse, children, grandchildren, other family members, friends and yourself. Deepen your understanding and your communication.

Next! The past is over. Rather you win or lose, move on. The next big adventure is now.

Over three quarters of Americans say they want to die at home, but only a quarter do. If you don't want to die in a **nursing home,** speak up!

Nuts. Eat a handful of **nuts** every day for health and longevity.

"A river passes through many countries and each claims it for its own. But there is only one river."
                    A Sufi saying

"That is why true paths are essentially one path—because there is only one Spirit, one breath, one life, one energy in the universe. It belongs to none of us and all of us."
                    --Mathew Fox

"We credit scarcely any persons with good sense except those who are of our opinion."
                    --La Rochefoucauld

"I love everything that's old; old friends, old times, old manners, old books, old wines."
                    --Oliver Goldsmith

O

O stands for **openness.** Keep an open mind, listen to all views and don't jump to conclusions. Question your opinions and look for facts. Read, research, listen, reflect and ask questions, "Is this true? How do I know it is absolutely true? What are the facts vs. opinions, inferences, and assumptions? Who is the source? Am I biased?" Strive for open and honest communication. Learn to listen to various viewpoints. Be open to suggestions and concerns from family and friends. You don't have to act on them, but don't be stubborn or ornery about listening and weighing advice.

Opportunity. There are so many creative ideas, wonderful adventures, and meaningful work that can enrich your life at any age. Always wanted to own a Bed & Breakfast? Visit one close by and see if you can help by inn sitting, gardening, or checking in guests. You will meet so many wonderful people and feel useful and productive. Wanted to be a doctor when you were young but your parents thought you should marry instead and become a teacher? Volunteer at a hospital, nursing home, Hospice. No. You won't be doing surgery, but you'll be caring and comforting ill and dying people. Regret not playing a musical instrument or being in a play? Do it. You cannot go back and redo life, but there are countless opportunities to serve and be useful.

Oneness. As we mature, we see that we are related to everything and everyone. We are all part of that one great energy.

Optimism keeps you young. Cynicism makes you old.

Outrage is optional. You can strive to correct injustice and make the world better without anger. You can be for something and not against it.

Keep your mind **occupied** and stimulated with interesting thoughts.

Observe. Really look. See things fresh and clear.

"Prayer should be the key of the day and the lock of the night."
      --Thomas Fuller

"Peace starts within each one of us."
         --The Dalai Lama

"There never was a good war or a bad peace."
         --Benjamin Franklin

"That man is richest whose pleasures are the cheapest."
         --Henry David Thoreau

"Adopt the pace of nature, her secret is patience."
         --Ralph Waldo Emerson

"How poor are they that have not patience! What wound did ever heal but by degrees?"
         --William Shakespeare

P

P stands for **peace**. Do your best to be at peace with yourself and others. Getting along, understanding, and wishing everyone well is really the key to living with grace. Avoid conflict whenever possible. There are three things that will help to make your life less stressful: 1) Take less offense, 2) take things less personally and blame less, and 3) sometimes you just have to let things be. Make peace your intention.

Planning can prevent many problems. Make certain your home is safe. Use your creative and critical thinking skills to look into the future. If you live alone and have an extra room, you might want to consider a roommate. Having someone around can ease the loneliness, help with cost, and provide help in an emergency. When you need more help, you may be able to get live-in help and still have privacy. If you want to age in place, you have to **plan ahead**.

Prayer, mediation, contemplative quiet, stillness are a means to connect with our spiritual selves. Solitude can help the distracted mind that is preoccupied with problems. Sit quietly so you can hear that still voice inside. We can all live a life of **praise.**

Prevent falls by being screened for balance problems. You can do exercises to increase your balance. Keep your house clutter free, take up throw rugs, keep a night light on and increase your strength.

Past. The past is over. Don't make an alter of the past. Live fully every minute and dwell in the **present** moment.

Perspective. The mind becomes clearer as you gain perspective, learn from experiences, and gain wisdom. What will matter years from now? Take a deep breath and take another look to see if things are really that bad.

Play. Every day find something to do that is sheer fun.

Passion. As long as you're alive you simply must have passion.

"Then from a remote part of his soul, from the past of his tired life, he heard a sound."
        Hermann Hesse in Siddharta

"All man's miseries derive from not being able to sit quietly in a room alone."
        --Blaise Pascal (1623-1662)

"Real questioning has no method, no knowing—just wondering freely, vulnerably, what it is that actually happening inside and out. Not the word, not the idea of it, not the reaction to it, but the simple fact."
        --Toni Packer

"I'm armed with more than complete steel—the justice of my quarrel."
        --Christopher Marlowe

"Learn to be silent.
Let your
quiet mind
listen and absorb."
        --Pythagoras (580 B.C.-500 B.C.)

Q

Q stands for **quiet**. Find that still, quiet, calm place within and rest there often. When the world is busy, when conflict swirls around you, when you feel critical or defensive. Stop. Take a deep breath and return to quiet. Breathe slowly until you dwell in this place of stillness. This is the time to find ways to be content and joyful.

Question your feelings. If you feel sadness, **quietly** enter grief and transcend it. Hold on to nothing, don't deny, rehash or allow your mind to spin. Sit quietly and enter into the human experience of suffering or what Ram Dass called "fierce grace." In quiet stillness allow yourself to respond consciously and creatively to difficulties by sitting with the pain.

Question. Dispute irrational thoughts. Question your beliefs and opinions. Question your negative thoughts. Ask yourself, "Is it true? How do I know it is absolutely true? How do I feel when I believe these thoughts?

As you age, you may start to **question** the meaning and value of your life. Who will miss you when you're gone? Who will remember you? Do you have creative work to contribute? Welcome these questions as a wake-up call to re-vitalize your life and to enjoy simple pleasures.

Quit whining. Really, it is unpleasant and unnecessary. You are not special in your trials, challenges or suffering.

Be quick to build bridges, not walls. Be quick to forgive.

"Finish each day and be done with it. You have done what you could. Some blunders and absurdities have crept in; forget about them as soon as you can. Tomorrow is a new day. You shall begin it serenely and with too high a spirit to be encumbered with your old nonsense."
        Ralph Waldo Emerson

"Live all you can; it's a mistake not to."
  --Henry James

"Old age is like flying a plane through a storm. Once you are aboard there is nothing you can do"
  --Golda Meir

"Maybe what we say to each other is not so important after all, but just that we are alive together and present for each other as best we can be."
  --Annie Lamott

"I make the most of all that comes and the least of all that goes."
  --Sara Teasdale

R

R stands for **resourceful**. You can age in place and be independent longer If you are creative and resourceful. Be open with unusual ideas and explore many options. You may want to rent a room to a college student or single working person. You may want to convert the basement, attic, garage, or add on a separate small apartment for a caregiver to stay if necessary at one point. If you live in the country or have to drive everywhere, you may want to look at buying a rental where you could walk to the grocery, bank, shops, bus lines, library, etc. When the time comes for you to give up driving or you need more care, you'll be ready. Be resourceful even if you're not old and can manage fine right now. It is easier to get used to sharing your home or living in a duplex when you're 70 rather than 90. Remember, you have a **right** to live independently.

Regrets. If you live in the present and focus on creating a meaningful future, you will have little time to think about past regrets. Don't waste a minute with what would have or could have been. Live in the present.

Reconcile with loved ones or friends who you've had a disagreement or falling out. Be the first to reach out with a card or letter and wish the other person well, and move on. Find peace through right action.

Renew yourself with walks, exercise, quiet, music, gardening or meditation. Take naps.

Retirement. What would you do if you could do anything you want? Why not plan on living your dream in retirement? What lifestyle would you choose? How will you grow spiritually and emotionally during retirement?

Re-imagine the last third of your life. How do you want to live and serve?

Return to life. Grieve after a loss. Retreat. Then return to life.

Respect yourself. Treat yourself and others with dignity.

"The spirit of man is the candle of the Lord."
        --Proverbs

"When you cease to make a contribution, you begin to die."
        --Eleanor Roosevelt

"Death can come at any moment, in any way. We do not know what is in store tomorrow, or, whether there will be a tomorrow, or even a tonight. But still, we have the golden present. Now we are alive and kicking. What shall we do now? Love all, serve all.
        --Sri Swami Satchidananda

"Certain environments, certain modes of life, certain rules of conduct are more conducive to inner and outer harmony than others. There are, in fact, certain roads that one may follow. Simplification of life is one of them."
        --Anne Morrow Lindbergh

"For those who grow old, life is at its sweetest."
        Sophocles

"What can give us surer knowledge than our senses? With what else can we better distinguish the true from the false?"
        --Lucretius

"Pilgrimage to the place of the wise is to find escape from the flame of separateness."
        --Jalaluddin Rumi

S

S stands for **safety**. Start now to look at ways your house could be safer. Get rid of rugs that can slip. Install hand railings and bars in your shower and bathroom. Make your house safe, clutter free, and comfortable.

Service. Giving to others is what makes life meaningful. What can you do to serve your partner, your children and your family? What can you do to improve your community?

Use all your **senses to savor** life; smell your coffee, taste your food, arrange flowers, hear the sounds birds, feel the texture of nature, and drink in the sights of morning. The senses help us to realize how sweet life is and how fortunate we are to be alive. **Savor.**

Seize the day! Surround yourself with interesting books, delicious food, and wonderful friends and family. When you know your days are numbered, they become more precious and meaningful. Each day is yours to enjoy. Delight in the glory of each sunrise and give thanks to each sunset. Be sparked by new ideas.

Stay in touch. Write letters, email, call and use Facebook to stay in touch with old friends and new. Never lose your **sensitivity** to others.

Savor your life and all the blessings you enjoy. Savor the ways you've blessed others. Practice kindness as you sprinkle blessings on everyone.

Seek forgiveness and understanding. Unburden your heart from any resentment and be at peace with yourself and others.

Self-righteousness creates distance. If you are too passionate in your political or religious views, arrogance and contempt grow and you exclude and hurt others.

Smaller plates. Yes, something this simple works. Also, **eat slowly.**

"I can't help but think that at the end of your life, when you look back, there'll be a tone. And that tone will come from the essence of how you live your day-to-day—what you did in that between time—because that is really your life."
   --Richard Linklater, film director

"Our life is what our thoughts make it."
   --Marcus Aurelius

"May you live all the days of your life."
   Jonathan Swift

"Stories have to be told or they die, and when they die; we can't remember who we are or why we're here."
   --Sue Monk Kidd, author, *The Secret Life of Bees*

Everybody today seems to be in such a terrible rush, anxious for greater developments and greater riches and so on, so that children have very little time for their parents. Parents have very little time for each other, and in the home begins the disruption of the peace of the world."
   --Mother Teresa of Calcutta

"Be a lamp unto yourself—take only the Truth for your refuge"
   --The Buddha

T

T stands for **tone**. It is not just the words that you use; it is the tone. What is the tone of your life? What do your thoughts, beliefs, emotions, and actions add up to? How do people feel after being around you? Do they smile? Do they feel encouraged and supportive? Take time to reflect on how you greet each day. Do you think the universe is supportive and loving or cruel and unfair? Do you take responsibility for your thoughts and actions or do you blame others? If you come from a victim point it is difficult to be positive. Challenge negative, irrational thoughts and replace them with positive, optimistic messages. Do this consistently and you'll wear a path in your neurons and being positive will be a habit. Focus on the best in life and yourself. Don't fret over what you did wrong, but live in this moment.

Tactful. You don't have to give voice to every thought. Being authentic and clear does not give you license to be rude or hurt other's feelings. Be kind. When someone voices a view you disagree with, allow the person to finish the thought completely. Don't interrupt. If it is an outrageous comment, let it fall flat. If you must respond, try a comment that isn't attacking or sarcastic. Work at being real, but agreeable and congenial. Say thank you **often.**

Trust. Trust that voice that says, "Something's not quite right." Don't ever be pressured into buying something or investing in a scheme especially by someone over the phone or Internet. Don't ever give out your social security number or bank account over the phone. Do not give your credit card number unless you made the call to order. If someone calls you asking for sensitive information, take their number and tell them you will call them back. Before you do talk with a trusted friend, attorney, banker or an adult child. Crooks can be very charming and sound legitimate. Pause before you act and be skeptical, cautious, and careful. See life as it is.

Telling your life story. Not only are you using mental skills, but you're passing on a priceless gift.

Time. Take time to pay attention, to savor life, and to appreciate each other. What is the rush? Have a nice cup of **tea.** Green tea is even better.

Tapping. Use the proven method of tapping to help you focus, relax and reduce anxiety. It all starts with loving and accepting yourself.

Tai Chi is a series of gentle flowing movements that promote health and mental relaxation. It is a movement meditation.

"Your pain has a story. Listen to it rather than try to shelve or push through it."
        -Kristen Munson

"You can love completely without complete understanding."
        --Norman Maclean,
        A River Runs Through it

"Treat people as if they were what they should be, and you help them become what they are capable of becoming."
        --Goethe

"The unexamined life is not worth living."
        --Socrates

"The afternoon of human life must also have a significance of its own and cannot be merely a pitiful appendage to life's morning.
        --Carl Jung

"If your heart were sincere and upright, every creature would be unto you a looking-glass of life and a book of holy doctrine."
        --Thomas A. Kempis

U

U stands for **understanding**. Seek to understand others rather than to simply press your point of view or opinion. Treat others with respect and a willingness to suspend judgment. Do the same with the big questions. At this stage in life, it is important to shift your focus from knowing to understanding and unraveling the mystery of life. Firm beliefs and dogma may have made you feel secure, but you are confident in your being now and can venture into unknown territory. Do you have **unexamined** beliefs, notions or opinions? Question, challenge yourself, use critical thinking, talk with people who have different beliefs and opinions. Listen. Stop ranting, stand back and observe.

Seek to **understand** the great mysteries of life. Carl Jung said that every question after fifty is a spiritual question. He stressed that as the physical energy wanes, spirituality becomes more important. Turn inward and contemplate the great mysteries of life and death. Read widely. Explore. Listen. Put aside your beliefs and keep an open mind.

Unconscious mind. Alan Watts once said that using only the conscious mind for perception and learning is like using a flashlight to see in an auditorium. The power of the unconscious mind to illumine is like lighting the auditorium with floodlights. When we switch off the mind we can get a glimpse of the **ultimate truth**. Sit quietly, meditate, pray, and simple be still. There is a universality of spirituality that can help create a richer life and true understanding of oneness.

Unsent letters. Write letters to people whom you have resentment, anger, or guilt. Tell them about your deepest feelings. Hold nothing back. You don't have to send them, in fact, you can burn them in a ceremony of forgiveness. Get your feelings out and then move on.

What **untapped possibilities** lie within you, just waiting to be born?

"A vain man may become proud and imagine himself pleasing to all when he is in reality a universal nuisance."
> --Spinoza

"To be a Sufi is to cease from taking trouble; and there is no greater trouble for thee than thine own self, for when thou art occupied with thyself, thou remainest away from God."
> --Abu Sa'id

"Project yourself into the probable future that will unfold with each choice that you are considering. See how you feel. Ask yourself, 'Is this what I really want?' And then decide."
> --Gary Zukav, author of The Seat of the Soul

"Things which matter most must never be at the mercy of things which matter least."
> --Goethe

"Have patience with all things, but chiefly have patience with yourself. Do no lose courage in considering your own imperfections, but instantly set about remedying them---every day begin the task anew."
> --Saint Francis De Sales

"Be a life long or short, its completeness depends on what it was lived for."
> David Starr Jordan

V

V stands for **vitality**. When you are curious, loving, kind, aware and healthy, you burst with vitality regardless of age. Music and the arts can at vitality and beauty to your life. Sing, dance, paint and create every day!

Values. What do you hold as sacred? This is the time to reflect of what values are most important for you and why. What values are most important for a thriving society? What ways can you pass these values on to the next generation? When you retire, you can do what you want. **Value** that free time.

Visualize. Imagine the kind of person you want to be at 100. What future do you want to create for yourself?

Vitamins are important and if you eat well, you'll get most of them from a good diet heavy on fruits and vegetables. However, most of us don't get enough Vitamin D. Ask your doctor if you should take vitamins.

Volunteer and get involved in the community. There are many ways to contribute your time, talents, and energy to service clubs or community projects. Volunteering improves mental outlook, reduces stress and increases longevity. You will also meet new people and gain a sense of satisfaction from knowing you have served your community. Just be careful that you don't fill every hour with busyness. Over activity can be one way of avoiding pain and grief. Carve out time to go within.

Vote as long as you're able and encourage young people to be informed and vote.

Vigorously embrace life.

Vanity is simply self-obsession.

"A man's name, title and rank are artificial and impermanent; they do nothing to reveal what he really is, even to himself."
--Jean Giraudoux

"Genius is one per cent inspiration and ninety-nine percent perspiration."
--Thomas Edison

"Selfishness is not living as one wishes to live, it is asking others to live as one wishes to live."
--Oscar Wilde

"The most revolutionary question is 'What do you want?'

--Alan Watts

"No wise man ever wished to be younger."
--Jonathan Swift

"With the ancient is wisdom; and in the length of days understanding."
--Book of Job

"Teach us to number our days aright, that we may gain a heart of wisdom."
--Psalm 90:12

W

W stands for getting it in **writing**. Go to your local hospital or doctor and ask for advance directives, which are legal documents to assure future health care choices. These documents let your doctor and other heath care providers know your wishes concerning medical treatment. You should have 1.) Instructions for healthcare (Living Will) and 2.) A Power of Attorney for Health Care. Keep these and other important documents in binder and make copies for each of your children. Talk about your end of life **wishes** and how you want to live and where documents are filed. There should be no confusion or misunderstanding. **What do you want?** You are not selfish for wanting to live in your own home and be as independent as possible.

Write. Consider writing your memoir or **write** a letter of love to your children, grandchildren and unborn great, great grandchildren. If you don't have children, write a letter to a young friend, relative or neighbor child.

Work. There is a deep pleasure in **work** and in making a contribution and feeling useful are important at every stage of life. Find something that engages your whole mind and body. Read, write, use your creative problem solving and balance your day with gardening, or woodworking.

Wake up. Too many people live their entire lives without really being aware. Growing older can give you time to really notice, to question, to study and create discipline. Now is the time to engage in truly living.

Wonder, joy, and curiosity keep you youthful.

Fine **wine** is a great metaphor for aging. It takes time to mellow and be truly excellent. **Wisdom** comes with experience and reflection.

Whole. Eat whole, satisfying foods that are **wholesome.**

Drink water with your meals.

"The entire sum of existence is the magic of being needed by just one person."
                Vi Putnam

"To exist is to co-exist."
                --Gavriel Marcel

"Exuberance is beauty."
                --William Blake

"To display his eternal attributes in their inexhaustible variety, the Lord make the green fields of time and space."
                --Jami

X

X stands for **crossing out** negative thoughts and complaints. There are really two kinds of people: Those who become more positive, open, kinder, and loving as they age and those who become more negative, picky, petty, and mean-spirited as they age. Look on life with appreciation and generosity. Find beauty everywhere, and give thanks that you're alive to enjoy the sheer **eXtravagance** of life. Denounce the notion that youth is king. Instead embrace the vast **eXperience**, the wisdom, the insights, and grace that aging brings. Stop pining for youth. What a waste of time.

Cross out perfection. There isn't much in life that demands perfection. There is no room for error if you're a surgeon or pilot, but cooking, gardening, writing, and art require only willingness. Relax. Jump in.

EXpressing your wishes and desires. Don't assume that your loved ones know what you want. Speak up! Tell people you appreciate them. Express gratitude for each day. Spend time with those you love. Get to know your neighbors and build communities. Don't isolate yourself. We **co-eXist** with other to help, support, and create meaningful lives. When all is said and done, we are all each other's brothers and sisters. We are all one.

EXperiment. Elders have a responsibility and the freedom to experiment with new ways of thinking and being. Test out new technology, new trends, new ways of relating to others to create peace and protect the earth. Elders have nothing to lose by being innovative and creative.

"To be seventy years young is sometimes far more cheerful and hopeful than to be forty years old."
        --Oliver Wendell Homes Jr.

"If we could see the miracle of a single flower clearly, our whole life would change."
        --Buddha

"For the unlearned, old age is winter; for the learned, it is the season of the harvest."
        Hasidic Proverb

"Everything that irritates us about others can lead us to an understanding of ourselves."
        --Carl G. Jung

"In talking with someone, does one realize how little we can actually know? How uncertain we are? How our yearning for a secure self gets frustrated and foiled time and time again? Can all the fears, pains, and doubts that accompany this shared work be deeply felt and seen together without giving way o any escapees?"
        -- Toni Packer

"Yoga brings together things that are seemingly apart. It brings together the body with the heart, mind, and soul. With yoga, we develop the capacity to listen to our bodies and become more sensitive to what it is saying."
        -Camille Litalien

Y

Y stands for a **youthful attitude**. Your higher self is ageless. You are not your body, your roles, circumstances, or possessions. **Stay young at heart** by being full of energy, vitality, curiosity, wonder, and love.

Yeah! You made it! Saying **yes** to life. Celebrate each birthday. You get to live another fabulous year. You don't need anyone's approval to say yes to life.

Yield. Surrender to what is and don't dwell on what was or could be. Listen to your body. If it wants you to slow down, slow down. If your body wants to take a nap, take a nap. Yield to what seems appropriate. Don't argue or struggle or as Aldous Huxley said, "Don't borrow trouble." Focus on what you can do and allow enjoyment in the moment.

It's not about **you.** You are not the target. Acknowledge that sometimes your feelings will be hurt, usually unintentionally. When you're self-absorbed, it is easy to be offended. Remind yourself that only your thoughts can hurt you. Choose to see the best in others and don't get caught up in believing that everything is about you. One of the advantages of aging is to loosen the effect of the ego.

Yoga is a philosophy that uses the body to connect with the mind and spirit. It can help you build strength and endurance and improves posture and balance. Listening to your breath is a transforming experience.

Ying/yang. As you age, you start to see the duality of life. An attachment in one extreme, causes a reaction in the opposite direction. Turn it around, and see inward. The world is a mirror, which reflects the self.

Yearning for meaning, belonging and connection. It's a life lesson worth learning; everyone wants support, not criticism. We want to belong.

"Nothing great was ever achieved without enthusiasm."
      --Ralph Waldo Emerson,
         American philosopher and poet

"Life is no brief candle to me. It is a sort of splendid torch which I've got hold of for the moment, and I want to make it burn as brightly as possible before handing it on o future generations."
      --George Bernard Shaw

The strongest and sweetest songs yet remain to be sung."
      -- Walt Whitman

"I shall grow old, but never lose life's zest,
Because the road's last turn will be the best."
      --Henry Van Dyke

Z

Z stands for **zest**. Appreciating life, enjoying simple pleasures, living in the present moment, delighting in people, being able to flow with changes, and bouncing back after inevitable losses are all important for living with exuberance. Live with enthusiasm. The best is yet to come.

Get your ZZZZZZZZZ's. The world would be changed for the better if people got more sleep and were more rested. There would be fewer accidents, less conflicts, less griping and complaining and more joy, peace, serenity, clarity and production. If you may find yourself having trouble falling to sleep or waking up in the night, try these tips:

- Prepare your body and mind for sleep.
- Turn off electronics (including TV) an hour or so before you sleep.
- Sleep in a dark room that is cool.
- Create a relaxing routine of meditation, or quiet time.
- Stop caffeine by lunch and don't drink any liquid after dinner.
- Exercise every day and try yoga.
- Eat dinner about three or four hours before you sleep.
- Try a natural herb such as melatonin, valerian root or chamomile.
- Have a routine like a warm bath or reading a relaxing book before bed.
- Use a fan or a sleep machine for white noise or wear ear-plugs.
- Go to bed earlier and get up earlier.
- Relax. Fretting only makes it worse. You can always take a nap.
- If you wake up, don't look at the clock.
- Be aware of how warm and comfortable you are and give thanks. Relax every muscle in your body and empty your mind of all thoughts.
- If you wake up, breathe slowly. Imagine that somewhere thousands of monks, nuns, priest, rabbis and people of every race and religion are meditating or praying. Join them.

Part Three:

References, Exercises, Quotes

"You can't learn from remembering. You can't learn from guessing. You can learn only from moving, forward at the rate you are moved, as brightness, into brightness."

-Sarah Manguso

"We are not yet what we shall be, but we are growing toward it."
　　　　--Martin Luther

"Just sit there right now
Don't do a thing
Just rest.

For your separation from God,
From love,

Is the hardest work
In this
World."
　　　　　　-Hafiz, 14th-century Sufi poet

EXERCISES

Exercise A: Visualize yourself as a wise, old sage and ask how you can be a more authentic person today.

Write about a recent incident where you were not as authentic as you would have liked to be. If you could time travel back, how would you handle it differently?

What lessons do you want to pass on to your loved ones about being authentic? What have you learned that would help others?

Exercise B: What beliefs support you? What beliefs sabotage you?

Write a letter to young person, let's say a granddaughter, telling her how much you believe and support her. Make a bucket list of things you want to do before you die.

Exercise C: Visualize yourself as a wise, old sage and ask how you could practice conscious living today? How can you be more mindful? Eat an orange slowly using all your senses. Pick out a tree and visit it every day or so. Notice the changes.

What barriers do you face in communicating with kindness and clarity? What situations are most difficult for you to be direct and assertive? If you could time travel back, how would you handle it differently? What have you learned that would help others?

What lessons do you want to pass on to your loved ones about being creative, flexible and open to change? What have you learned that would help others?

Exercise D: Write about ways you dispute negative thoughts. What helps you stay positive?

What have you discovered about life that has added meaning and joy?

Exercise E: When did you learn that you are good enough?

What do you do to increase your energy?

Estimate how many years you think you have left to live based on health, age and genes. Next, write out what you want to accomplish in those remaining years. These goals may be simple such as, "I want to sing more often."

Exercise F: Do you spend time worrying? What are your biggest fears? What can you do to face your fears?

Write about forgiveness. Have you forgiven yourself for past mistakes?

Exercise G: In what ways are you truly blessed? How do you show gratitude?

Goals: What are your three goals for aging? For example,
1. I want to be listened to and respected.
2. I want to be in control of my life, independent and make my own decisions.
3. I want to be healthy, happy, and peaceful.

Exercise H: What can you do to improve your health? Do you have a routine?
Write about happiness. Tell me about hurrying less.

Exercise I: What can you do today to be more independent in the future?

How can you get more involved in the community?

Write about good intentions. What happened?

Exercise J: Write about your journey. Sketch an illustration—a river or path that illustrates your life. Mark the top three big transitions.

Have you learned to be less judgmental?

What gives you great joy?

Exercise K: Write about kindness. When did you learn that it was important? How do you practice kindness?

Exercise L: Write about laughter. When was the last time you had a good laugh? Who makes you laugh? Do you laugh more than rant?

Letters of Love: Consider writing a simple letter of love to your spouse, children, grandchildren, special nieces or nephews, special friends, etc.

Mind map: Part A. On a blank piece of paper, write the word **LESS** in the middle of the paper and circle it. Draw spokes from this main word and jot down all the things you want less of in your life. For example, you might write the words stress, worry, aches and pain, tension, etc.

Exercise M: Tell me about marriage. What has it meant to you? What advice would you give to a young couple?

What is magical to you?

Play with a baby or young child. What magical things happen when you're playful?

Mind map: Part B. Turn over the paper marked LESS (see mind map part A under L). Write the word MORE in the center of the page and around it jot down all the things you want more of in your life. For example, you might write the words peace, health, kindness, understanding, etc. Share this exercise with others and discuss what you want more and less of in your life. Now write out a plan for how to work on being more fulfilled.

Exercise N: Write to me about the word, notice. What do you do to increase your awareness? What could you do now, instead of waiting?

How do you focus on the present moment and keep enthused about tomorrow?

Exercise O: How did you learn to be open to new ideas, friends, and the mysteries of life?
What would you say to a young person about being open-minded?

Exercise P: How do you plan to age in place? What can you do today to be safer, healthier, and more independent? How are you powerful?

Exercise Q: Do you spend a part of each day in quiet? What has stillness taught you?

Are you Quick to forgive? Do you ask questions of others?

Questions: Thousands of years ago, the Delphi said that there are three universal questions that concern all of mankind. Reflect on these and other philosophical questions.

Who am I?
What is my purpose?
What will become of me?

What is your place in the universe?
What you believe about God?
What do you believe about the afterlife?
What books have you read that have helped you to clarify your views?
How would you describe a perfect day?
If you could do anything and age, money and health were not factors, what would you do?

Exercise R: In what ways are you resourceful? Do you have trouble asking for help? Do you take pleasure in reading? Write about regrets.

What do you realize is more important than you thought when you were younger?

Re-imagine what the rest of your life will be. Describe how your will continue to grow, serve, work and relate to others.

Exercise S: Write about your spiritual life.

How have you slowed down?

Write about siblings. Do you have a good relationship? Write about sharing.

Keep it simple. When you start to complain, remember:

> It's really not that complicated:
> - Approach each day with a gentle, welcoming, positive, joyous, grateful and upbeat tone. Engage.
> - Look for the best in others and in life. Embrace.
> - Have fun. Life isn't about fighting, enduring, and surviving the storms; it is about dancing in the rain. Dance.

Exercise T: Write about being tactful. What sayings do you use to avoid confrontation? For example: "That's one way of looking at it." Or "I respect your viewpoint, but I see things differently." or "What experiences help form that perception or way of thinking?"

Write about being thoughtful and sensitive. How do you balance being authentic and truthful and kind and tactful?
Write about trust. Are you too trusting?

Do you strive to be authentic and tell the truth? Are your relationships strong enough to endure honesty and anger? Robert Raines refers to this honesty as, "Anger can sometimes be the friend of intimacy in a family relationship where both parties to a quarrel care enough to hang on until a mutually agreeable solution emerges." Write about your disagreements with siblings or other family members.

Exercise U: Write about understanding. How do you show your understanding of others? Do you love unconditionally? Tell me what unexamined beliefs you have inherited or acquired?

Exercise V: How do you increase your vitality? What makes you feel alive?

Visualize yourself as a 100-year-old elder. Describe your wise, kind and spiritual self. How do you look, walk, talk and act? What happened to create this magnificent person? Describe the tone and energy flowing from you.

What advice does your elder give to you for living the last third of your life?

What would your wise old elder say to you now about being understanding and loving?

Exercise W: Do you have the willingness to live consciously and grow emotionally? Ho do you recapture wonder and see life fresh through the eyes of a child? Instead of blame or regret, do you say, "What can I learn from this?"

Whom do you need to forgive?

Whom do you need to ask for forgiveness?

Exercise X: How do you express your truth? How do you express love, warmth, interests?

Exercise Y: Do you yearn for more connection, a sense of belonging, purpose? Write to me about longing.

How do you say "yes" to life?

Exercise Z: What routine works for you to get enough sleep? How do you relax and feel rested and ready for a new day? For example,
* I take a warm bath.
* I read before bed.
* I don't worry or fret. I just relax my body and meditate if I wake in the night.

In what ways do you have a zest for life? How do you act zany?

Take Ten: The Ten-Minute Exercise Program

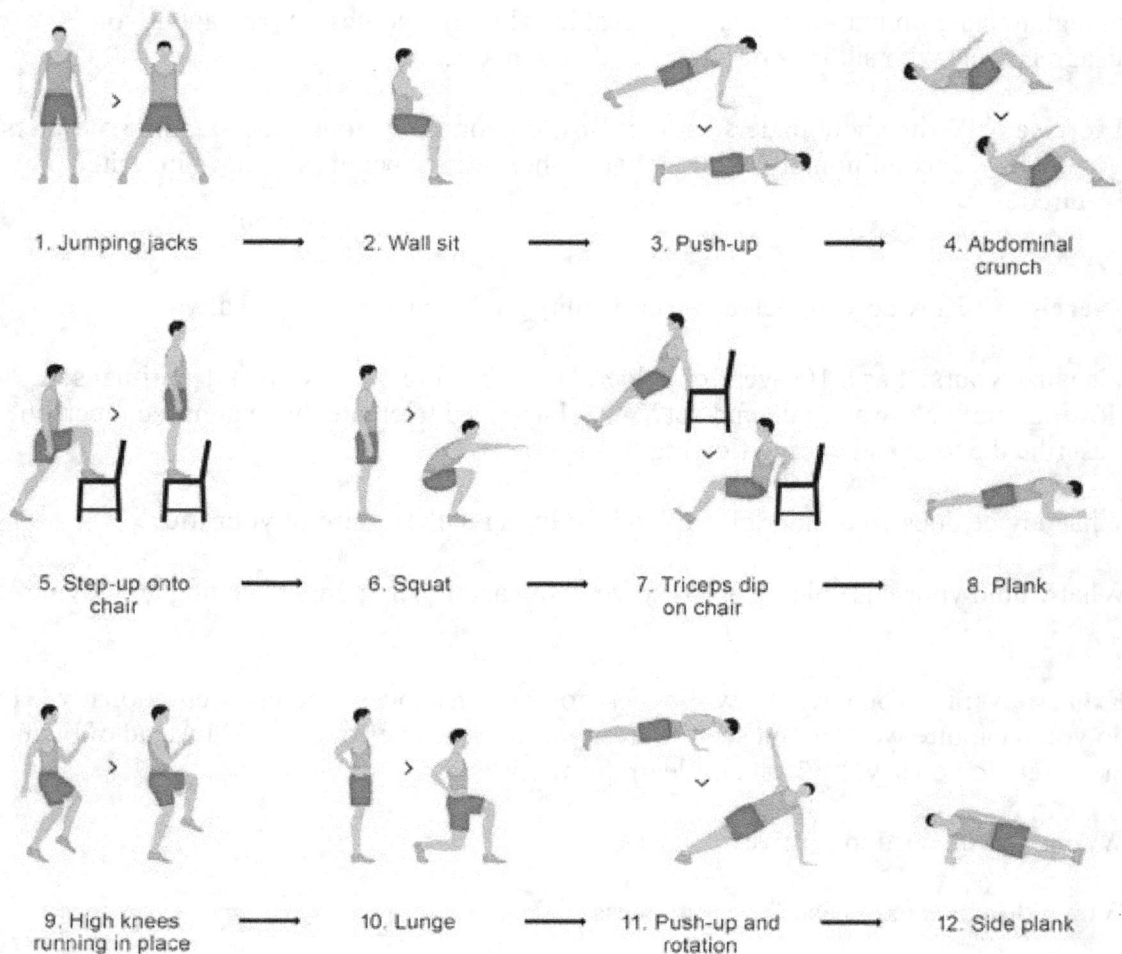

Yoga, Tai Chi and Stretching

You can integrate a stretching program with the above exercises. Create one that works for you. Here's an example:

1. **Jumping jacks and wall sit.**
2. **Neck and shoulder mobility**. Reach to the sky. Stretch. Scrunch shoulders and relax. **Clock** and you stretch arms and circle around. Stretch your fingers and circle your wrist. Hug arms and clean a table and mirror. Lift arms as you do tai chi movements.
3. **Back and forth as you squat, lunge and lift knees high**.
4. **Plies** with lateral stretch. Lift your heel as you come up.
5. **Heel and ankle stretches** as you lean into a chair or kitchen cabinet or sink. Lift your heels as you exercise your ankles, lift separately and together as you hold onto a chair or counter. Move and crunch your toes. Stretch your ankles left and right and flex and point.
6. **Sit ups** with slow leg extensions. Finish with **bridge.**
7. **Lift legs** and draw circles and stretch bringing one leg over. Rock.
8. On all fours do pushups, rotation, and **cat stretch and lion's stretch.**
9. **Opposite Arm and Leg extensions** on all fours.
10. **Child's pose** as you stretch ankles and go to each side.
11. **Side plank for count of 8, lift leg, straighten, bring leg over.**
12. **Stretch one leg out and touch, wave leg and bend 3 times as you stretch out in front.**
13. **Spine stretches.** Sit and stretch hips, put hands under raised knees. Move back and forth. Legs out in front, bring one over to side and stretch spine as you left and stretch neck Reach over with arms.
14. **Triceps dip on chair and leg stretches on chair. Bend leg.**
15. **Balance exercises. Alphabet with legs extended and flexed.**
16. **Warriors poise, then prayer pose on one foot.**

Finish with affirmations: I am Enough.
                                 I am Whole.
                                 I am Blessed. I am.

Low Carb Dinners

Slow Cooker Lemon Olive Chicken

Serves 6 to 8
- 2 cups chopped onions
- 8 skinless chicken thighs (bone-in or boneless)
- 1 lemon, thinly sliced and seeded
- 1 cup green olives, pitted
- 1 Tbsp. white-wine vinegar
- 2 tsp. herbes de Provence
- 1 bay leaf
- 1/2 tsp. kosher salt
- 1 tsp. freshly ground black pepper
- 1 cup chicken stock
- 1/2 cup chopped, fresh flat-leaf parsley

Arrange the onions in the bottom of a slow cooker and top with the chicken thighs. Place a lemon slice on each thigh. Add the olives, vinegar, herbs de Provence, bay leaf, salt, pepper and chicken stock. Cook on low heat for 5 to 6 hours. Remove and discard the bay leaf. Serve each portion sprinkled with the chopped parsley

Cassoulet

- Low-calorie cooking-oil spray
- 1 pound lean pork, diced
- 3 ounces chorizo sausage, sliced
- 1 onion, chopped
- 3 garlic cloves, minced
- 1 red bell pepper, cored, seeded and diced
- 2 celery stalks, sliced
- 1 carrot, diced
- 2 cups tomato purée
- 1 tsp. dried Mediterranean herbs
- 2 (14-ounce) cans cannellini beans, drained

Directions: Preheat the slow cooker. Spray a large skillet with a little low-calorie cooking-oil spray and place over high heat until hot. Add the pork, a few pieces at a time, until all the meat is in the pan and cook for 5 minutes, stirring, until browned. Use a slotted spoon to transfer the pork to the slow-cooker pot.

Add the chorizo and onion to the skillet and cook for 4 to 5 minutes, until the onion has softened. Stir in the garlic, red bell pepper, celery, carrot, tomato purée and herbs. Season to taste and bring to a boil, stirring.

Place the beans in the slow-cooker pot, pour in the tomato purée mixture and stir well. Level the surface with the back of a spoon, then scatter the bread crumbs evenly over the top. Cover and cook on low for 8 to 10 hours, until the pork is tender. Spoon into shallow bowls and serve with a salad, if you like.

Poached Salmon

Serves 6
Ingredients
- 1 medium onion, thinly sliced
- 1 medium carrot, thinly sliced
- 1 celery rib, thinly sliced
- 6 whole black peppercorns
- 1 bay leaf
- 1 large fresh flat-leaf parsley sprig
- Salt
- 3 Tbsp. white wine vinegar
- 2 cups water
- 6 salmon steaks, at least 1 inch thick
- Freshly ground pepper

In a large slow cooker, combine the onion, carrot, celery, peppercorns, bay leaf, parsley, a pinch of salt, the vinegar, and the water. Cover and cook on high for 2 hours.

Sprinkle the salmon steaks with salt and pepper to taste and place them in the cooker.

Spoon some of the liquid over the top. Cover and cook on high for 30 minutes, or until done to taste.

Tips:

1. Use a smaller plate.
2. Drink water or hot tea with your meals and eat slowly.
3. Fill your plate with salad, veggies, protein and a little fruit.

Journal and Discussion Questions

Write out your typical day and look for ways to make small positive changes. How do you start your day? What would you like to change?

Here is How I Start My Day

I wake up without an alarm clock. I give thanks for the day and smile. I ask for guidance: *"Let me be attentive and fully aware. If there is something you want me to do, let me wake up to this purpose. Show me, without any misunderstanding, that this intuition, this nudge is coming from Spirit and not my ego. Allow my creativity to flow and help me to be aware of sparks of genius and to act on them. Allow inspiration to help me to rebound from discouragement or failure. My intention is to be useful, kind and focused throughout the day. Let me see the beauty all around. Let me know my purpose.*

Typical day: I mediate for about 15 minutes. Then I get up and drink a glass of water with apple cider vinegar and one without. I have black coffee with a variety of fruit including one prune (helpful for bone density). I do my basic exercise and stretches for a half hour and tap.

Sam and I take a rigorous hour walk with our dogs everyday. Then I eat a banana with peanut butter and enjoy a latte made with coffee, soy, almond and skim milk sprinkled with cocoa and cinnamon. I take a multiple vitamin, plus Vit D and baby aspirin, and a Ts of fermented foods and a probiotic. I sit down and write for an hour most days or garden or take care of grandchildren. I have an early lunch of either egg or tuna salad or soup. have green tea. After lunch, I sit quietly for about 20 minutes and meditate. Sometimes I'll read or take a short nap. In the afternoon, I switch to several cups of decaf green tea and have a piece of dark chocolate and a handful of nuts. I try to eat around 5 or no later than 6. And have a big salad and fish or chicken including a variety of vegetables and a big cup of chamomile tea. Then I stop drinking for the night. I have a one small glass of wine when out with friends a few times a week. Once a week or so, I'll have sour dough bread and pasta and dessert. I never drink soda or juice except POM once a week with popcorn. Before bed, I stretch and do kettle ball. I take a magnesium, calcium and zinc supplement and a melatonin.

Around 9, I un-plug and take a warm bath. I go to bed around 9:30 and then read until around 10. Our bedroom is dark, cool, and has a fan for background noise. I usually sleep until around 5:00 or 5:30. If I do wake up in the night, I don't look at the clock. Instead I meditate and if necessary, take a melatonin. I usually sleep well and wake up refreshed and ready for a full day. That's my day. Not terribly exciting, but busy and very satisfying. I often care for my grandchildren and we play and laugh. I love our cats and dogs, I feel unconditional love from them and an amazing energy that makes me happy. I help in my grandchildren's classrooms for an hour or so one day a week, sit on a few community boards, and sing in a group once or twice a month. In general, I feel useful, happy and grateful. I meet for tea with several girlfriends often and value my friends and family. In the summer, I garden for hours a week. When I have a deadline, I write for hours every day, but I get up and stretch often. I'm content and fulfilled and doing what I enjoy most. I retired from a full-time university position, but I still write, teach and Sam and I run a bed and breakfast inn, so we are not retired, but we do have flexibility.

What I'd like to change: *I'd like to have more free time and more help with gardening and cleaning. I'd like to get fully organized. I'd like to have a regular writing schedule. I'd like to take more time on my appearance, dress more elegant and keep up with fashion. I generally wear what is really comfortable and can go months without a haircut. I'd like to laugh more and spend more time with good friends. Right now, my young grandchildren need me and I adore them. They care that I'm attentive, kind and fun. They don't care what I wear or if my hair is styled. So, my priorities seem obvious and important. Change will come and I'll have free time and no regrets that I didn't spend time with family. We have a strong bond.*

The Rest of Your Life…..

Estimate how many years you think you'll have left. How do you want to live? What do you want to do the rest of your life?

This was an interesting exercise. Here's what I wrote: *I plan on living another thirty years or so. I want to continue to spend a lot of time with my family. I'd like to take an hour walk every morning after a cup of good coffee and the morning paper. I want to be writing books and teaching classes and workshops. I want quiet evenings with Sam. That would include savoring a nice dinner with wine and dessert and evenings reading and watching our favorite shows and movies. I want to enjoy good friends, eating out and cooking for each other. I want to be in a book club and discuss interesting books. I want to continue to enjoy our children, grandchildren, and hopefully great grandchildren. I would like to support and help them with travel and education. I want the time to really get to know each of them well. I would like to live in a nice home with lovely surroundings. I would like a young person to live in a detached studio to help with yard work and cleaning. I expect to garden and tend my roses. I will sing and read poetry daily. I plan on being involved in church and spiritually active groups. Sam and I will travel as much as we feel comfortable and will continue to go back to Michigan to see family and friends and enjoy our lake cottage. I want to study aging and death and dying. I want a conscious death at home surrounded by my dear family. I could die in the beach house watching the ocean or die in my bed in the Victorian overlooking the rose garden.*

Reflect on some of the following themes. Write your thoughts in your journal and discuss with others.

Take Control: If you want to live long and well, it helps if you have good genes. However, research has shown that your behaviors, lifestyle, and habits play a large part in how successfully you age. By following a few simple guidelines, you can promote optimal health, increase energy and strength, maintain a healthy weight, be happier, sleep well and gain a greater sense of well being. Take control of what you can do to make positive changes in your life. It's really not that complicated—create healthy eating habits, exercise, trust your inner wisdom, and follow the gentle path of your wise sage.

Aging: Think about what your experience has been with aging people. Write about your grandparents or parents and their experiences. Tell me about your fears. Tell me about your wishes. How would you like to age? How would you like to die?

Beliefs: What beliefs do you have about aging? How have these beliefs changed over the years? Do you like your life now? How old do you feel inside? As Satchel Paige, the black baseball legend, asked, "How old would you be if you didn't know how old you were?"

Health: Describe your health. What do you do to improve your health? What are a few simple habits you've adopted that have made a difference in your health? What could you do to make positive changes? What is keeping you from being healthier?

Purpose: Determine what you want out of life. What is your life's purpose? How would you like to be remembered? Will your life have made a difference? Where do you find meaning and a sense of purpose? If you knew you would live forever, what would you do? If you knew you would die within a year, what would you do? Do you want to stay in your own home and be independent? Describe your life as a 90-year-old. Where will you be living?

Plans: How do your plans support your purpose? What plans do you have for the future? What is on your bucket list? Do you want to live independently as long as possible? If so, what plans have you made to make this goal a reality? Do you want to be as healthy and strong as possible? If so, what habits do you do on a daily basis that supports good health? Do you have enough money to live comfortably in old age? Do you have a living will set up? Have you talked with a financial advisor? Who will help support and care for you, if necessary? What plans can you put in place right now to live long and well?

Relationships: Describe your closest relationships. How could you improve them? Would you like more frequent contact and communication, more physical expressions of love, more time, or authentic and real communication? Be as specific as possible about what you want. Would you like to make more new friends? Would you like to deepen your relationships with old friends?

Forgiveness: Do you carry resentment or anger? Is there a grievance story that you tell yourself over and over? Is there someone with whom you have a conflict? Have you forgiven people who have hurt you? Have you asked for forgiveness from people whom you hurt? Do you wish everyone good will? Would you prefer to be right or have peace?

Know yourself: Take time to reflect on who you are and what you want. Gather pictures of yourself at various ages. Who was that sweet baby? Who was that three0year old? Describe your first five years. What is your birth order? Where did you live? Who took care of you? Where did you go to school? What were the major transitions in each decade of your life? What were your youthful dreams? How did you get from there to here?

Courage: It takes courage to rebound from loss and reinvent your life again and again. What gives you courage? When were you courageous? Whom do you admire for their courage? Where did you learn resiliency?

Documents

You will want to have a three -ring binder for all your documents and basic information. Keep it either filed or on your bookshelf in plain sight. Tell and show all your loved ones where this binder is kept. You will want it to be easily accessible and update it every year. One of the best gifts you can give your loved ones is the gift of simplicity. If you have taken care of your health directives, planned your funeral, and taken care of end-of-life issues, you will leave a blessing for your loved ones. There will not be questions about what you would have wanted or endless searching for documents. Tell your loved ones where you keep your address book (update it each year). The following are simple steps to take to get organized. Complete each of these headings:

Basic Information

Name   Place of Birth
Social Security Number
Important papers or certificates
 *Marriage license
 * Divorce papers
 * Military service
Computer pass word
Cell number
ATM
Current bills and receipts
Warranties
Insurance papers
Health Information
 *Primary care physician phone
 *Dentist   phone
 *Health Insurance copy of card
 *Hospital phone

    Credit cards   number and phone
Location of will
Hospice number

Basic Information upon my death

People to notify (list name, phone, email)
*Siblings and other family members
* Friends
*Minister
*Executor/Trustee
*Attorney
*Financial advisor
* Veterinarian (arrangements for pets)
* Accountant
* others: Guardians for children, hair dresser, gardener, etc.

Assets and their locations. List:
Safety Deposit Box   Location of key
Property, loans, deeds
Cars, boats, registration
Bank accounts, location, passwords
Insurance policies
Investments
Pension information
Income taxes and returns
Debts

Personal Property (you may want to take pictures of furniture, jewelry, art, and other assets). Write down where each asset came from and where you want it to go. You may want to explain why. Some people put post-it notes on the back of paintings, etc. It is a good idea to talk with your loved ones about your wishes now and how you are attempting to be fair and equal in your distribution. Reduce or eliminate hurt feelings by clear communications. For example, Mahogany chest with mirror. This was my mother's beloved chest and came with my parents when they traveled west. Give to Emily. She has always liked it and it will look perfect in her house.

End of Life Choices
Advance Directives are legal documents to assure future health care choices. They include 1). Instructions for Health Care (Living Will) and 2). Power of Attorney for Health Care. You have the right to give instructions about your own health care. This is called a **Living Will.** This is a document which tells your doctor and other health care providers whether or not you want life-sustaining treatments or procedures administered to you if you are in a terminal condition or a permanent unconscious state. It is called a "living will" because it takes effect while you are still living. State and federal law give

every competent adult, 18 years or older, the right to make their own health care decisions, including the right to decide what medical care or treatment to accept, reject or discontinue. If you do not want to receive certain types of treatment you have the right to make these wishes known.

The Advance Health Care Directive Form also includes a legal document which allows you appoint another person to make medical decision for you if you should become temporarily or permanently unable to make decisions for yourself. This is called a **Power of Attorney for Health Care.** This is a serious decision. You should select a person or persons who understand your wishes, values and whom you have trust and confidence. In addition to putting it in writing, you should tell all family members of your decision. (One woman had signed papers right after her husband died. She was in deep grief and ill. She forgot about this event and didn't think about it again until her children put her in a nursing home. The children whose names were not listed as having power of attorney had never seen the document or heard that it even existed). These stories are more common than you could ever imagine. Don't let this happen to you. This is an extremely important section of your documents. Communication is the key. You have the right to change or revoke your Advance Health Care Directive at any time. Each state will have a different form which you can obtain at your local hospital or from your physician. If you have questions speak to a Chaplain or Social Worker at the hospital. It is important that you discuss and give copies of advanced directives to your family, doctor, lawyer, and clergy. There should be no surprises about your wishes. The Advance Directive Form not only lets you write down your wishes about Power of Attorney, instructions for health care, but also includes a section on donation of organs and the selection of your primary physician. In most states, this form will be valid if it is signed by two qualified adult witnesses who are personally known to you and who are present when you sign or acknowledge your signature or it is acknowledged before a notary public in the state. Wallet cards are also available. For more information visit:
www.advdir.com
www.agingwithdignity.org
www.finalchoices.org

Wills and Living Trust. It is important to see an attorney who specializes in wills and living trusts. These are financial documents which allow you to plan for the distribution of your financial assets and property after your death. You can also discuss planned giving with your attorney. Don't put this off. The peace of mind this brings is worth every penny.

Obituary. In your binder, write a draft of your obituary. This is your opportunity to have your life presented as you want it to be. This will save your family a lot of time and confusion at a difficult time. You will know that dates, colleges, employment and all information that you want included is correct. One woman's obituary excluded her second husband and step -children because a daughter who wrote it didn't like her mother's second husband. Write a first draft, review and update every year or so (survivors can fill in date, location and cause of death). Here's basic information:

Name   Date and place of birth
Parent's name
Schools and universities attended, special honors or awards
Career information and highlights/Military service
Professional memberships, organizations/volunteer
Hobbies and passions
Survived by parents, siblings, spouse, children, grandchildren (list all names)
Preceded in death by parents, siblings, spouse, children, etc. (list all names).
Church attended
Time and place for viewings, wakes, services, memorial
Preferred donations to favorite charities instead of flowers

Planning Your Funeral or Memorial. Make your wishes known by considering the following:
What do you want done—burial or cremation? What kind of casket? Open or closed?
Where do you want to have a funeral or memorial? Place? Church, Funeral home, other.
Who do you want to officiate?
Where do you want to be buried or ashes scattered?
When –within days or at a time which is more convenient for family or congregation?
How do you want your service to look?
What tone do you want your service to have?
Program, bulletin, cards
   Songs, hymns, music, musician
   Psalms, readings, poems or quotes
   Slide show or pictures on display
   Flowers
   Ushers/pallbearers
   Who should speak?   Open mike?
   Eucharist?
   Reception or lunch?
Arrangements for body or organ donation
In a nutshell, give thought and express to your loved ones and write out your wishes.
What legacy do you want to leave?

Poems, Stories, Quotes

Include your favorite poems or quotes:

"I got out of bed
On two strong legs.
It might have been

Otherwise.
I ate
Cereal, sweet
Milk, ripe, flawless
Peach. It might
Have been otherwise.
I took the dog uphill
To the birch wood.
All morning I did
The work I love.
At noon I lay down
With my mate. It might
Have been otherwise.
We ate dinner together
At a table with silver
Candlesticks. It might
Have been otherwise.
I slept in a bed
In a room with paintings
On the walls, and
Planned another day
Just like this day.
But one day, I know,
It will be otherwise."
  --Jane Kenyon

My Children Are Coming Today

My children are coming today. They mean well. But they worry.
They think I should have a railing in the hall. A
telephone in the kitchen. They want someone
to come in when I take a bath.
They really don't like my living alone.
Help me to be grateful for their concern. And
help them to understand that I have to do
what I can as long as I can.
They're right when they say there are risks. I
might fall. I might leave the stove on. But there is
no challenge, no possibility of
triumph, no real aliveness without risk.
When they were young and climbed trees and
rode bicycles and went away to camp, I was

terrified. But I let them go.
Because to hold them would have hurt them.
Now our roles are reversed. Help them see.
Keep me from being grim or stubborn about it.
But don't let me let them smother me.

Green Winter, by E. Maclay, New York. Reader's Digest Press

"...from cradle to tomb, it's not that long a stay."
    --From the Musical Cabaret

"Let yourself be silently drawn by the strange pull of what you really love. It will not lead you astray."
    --Jalaluddin Rumi

If I Had My Life to Live Over
  --Nadine Stair

I'd dare to make more mistakes next time. I'd relax, I would limber up. I would be sillier than I have been on this trip. I would take fewer things seriously. I would take more chances. I would climb more mountains and swim more rivers. I would eat more ice cream and less beans. I would perhaps have more actual troubles, but I'd have fewer imaginary ones. You see, I'm one of those people who live sensibly and sanely hour after hour, day after day. Oh. I've had my moments, and if I had it to do over again, I'd have more of them. In fact, I'd try to have nothing else. Just moments, one after another, instead of living so many years ahead of each day. I've been one of those persons who never goes anywhere without a thermometer, a hot water bottle, a raincoat, and a parachute. If I had to do it again, I would travel lighter than I have.

If had my life to live over, I would start barefoot earlier in the spring and stay that way later in the fall. I would go to more dances. I would ride more merry-go-rounds. I would pick more daisies.

This is how the story goes....

The first day of school our professor introduced himself and challenged us to get to know someone we didn't already know. I stood up to look around when a gentle hand touched my shoulder.

I turned around to find a wrinkled, little old lady beaming up at me with a smile that lit up her entire being.

She said, 'Hi handsome. My name is Rose. I'm eighty-seven years old. Can I give you a hug?'

I laughed and enthusiastically responded, 'Of course you may!' and she gave me a giant squeeze.

'Why are you in college at such a young, innocent age?' I asked.

She jokingly replied, 'I'm here to meet a rich husband, get married, and have a couple of kids...'

'No seriously,' I asked. I was curious what may have motivated her to be taking on this challenge at her age.

'I always dreamed of having a college education and now I'm getting one!' she told me.

After class we walked to the student union building and shared a chocolate milkshake.

We became instant friends. Every day for the next three months we would leave class together and talk nonstop. I was always mesmerized listening to this 'time machine' as she shared her wisdom and experience with me.

Over the course of the year, Rose became a campus icon and she easily made friends wherever she went. She loved to dress up and loved the attention bestowed upon her from the other students. She was living it up. At the end of the semester we invited Rose to speak at our football banquet I'll never forget what she taught us. She was introduced and stepped up to the podium. As she began to deliver her prepared speech, she dropped her three by five cards on the floor. Frustrated and a little embarrassed she leaned into the microphone and simply said, 'I'm sorry I'm so jittery. I gave up beer for Lent and this whiskey is killing me! I'll never get my speech back in order so let me just tell you what I know.' As we laughed she cleared her throat and began, ' We do not stop playing because we are old; we grow old because we stop playing.

There are only four secrets to staying young, being happy, and achieving success. You have to laugh and find humor every day. You've got to have a dream. When you lose your dreams, you die. We have so many people walking around who are dead and don't even know it! There is a huge difference between growing older and growing up.

If you are nineteen years old and lie in bed for one full year and don't do one productive thing, you will turn twenty years old. If I am eighty-seven years old and stay in bed for a year and never do anything I will turn eighty-eight. Anybody! Can grow older. That doesn't take any talent or ability. The idea is to grow up by always finding opportunity in change. Have no regrets. The elderly usually don't have regrets for what we did, but rather for things we did not do. The only people who fear death are those with regrets.
'
She challenged each of us to study the lyrics and live them out in our daily lives. At the year's end Rose finished the college degree she had begun all those months ago.

One week after graduation Rose died peacefully in her sleep.

Suggested Readings

Allegra, Suzy: *How to Be Ageless*
Arrien, Angeles: *The Second Half of Life*
Bartocci, Barbara: *Midlife Awakenings*
Bolen, Jean: *Crones Don't Whine*
Butler, Katy: *Knocking on Heaven's Door*
Callanan, Maggie: *Final Gifts*
Carlson, Richard and Kristine: *If You Had an Hour to Live*
Carter, Jimmy: *The Virtues of Aging*
Crowley, Chris: *Younger Next Year*
Dyer, Wayne: *Wisdom of the Ages*
Ellis, Neeah: *If I Live to be 100*
Hansen, Mark Victor: *How to Make the Rest of Your Life the Best of Your Life*
Hibner, Dixie: *Aging with Enthusiasm, race and Dignity*
Hough, Arthur: *Facing Age Squarely*
Lawrence-Lihtfoot, Sara: *The Third Chapter*
Latimer, Rebecca: *You're Not Old Until You're Ninety*
Lee, Grace: *On the Way to Over the Hill*
Packer, Toni: *The Work of This Moment*
Pipher, Mary: *Another Country: Navigating the Emotional Terrain of Our Elders*
Raines, Robert: *A Time to Live: Seven Steps of Creative Aging*
Robbins, John: *Healthy at 100*
Rubin, Lillian: *Women of a Certain Age*
Sahn, Jennifer: *Thirty Year Plan*
Schachter-Shalomi, Zalman: *From Age-ing to Sage-ing*
Snelling, Lauraine: *100 Good Things That Happen As You Grow Older*
Stein, Murray: *In Midlife*
Sullender, Scott: *Losses in Later Life*
Watson, Elizabeth: *Guests of My Life*
Voorhees, Randy: *Old Age is Always 15 Years Older Than I Am*

About the Authors

Sharon K. Ferrett has over forty-five years of experience in higher education as a college and university dean, director, professor and academic advisor. Her books include: *Peak Performance*, tenth edition (McGraw-Hill, 2014), *Positive Attitudes at Work* (Irwin, 1994), *Strategies: College and Career Success* (Irwin 1996). *Getting and Keeping the Job You Want,* second edition (Irwin, 1995). Her presentations include: forgiveness, student success, motivation, writing memoir, creativity, working with difficult people, and health and wellness.

Sharon earned her B.A. and M.A. in communication from Western Michigan University and a Ph.D. in higher education administration and organizational communication from Michigan State University. She also did graduate work at the University of Michigan, University of Edinburgh and University of London. You can reach her at **sharonferrett@gmail.com**.

Sarah A. Bourque is a science and mathematics teacher at Sunnybrae Middle School. She is passionate about helping students learn healthy habits, to manage stress, and to love learning. Her writing and workshops include student success, bullying, empathy, and health and wellness. She practices yoga, loves to hike, and paddleboard. Sarah earned her B.A.in communication and M.A. in education from California State University, Chico and a teaching credential from Humboldt State University. She also studied in Italy for a year. You can reach her at sarahpennisi@gmail.com.

Never doubt that a small group of thoughtful committed citizens can change the world. Indeed, it is the only thing that ever has.

MARGARET MEAD